cancerproof

your body

ROSS HORNE

cancerproof
your body

Angus&Robertson
An imprint of HarperCollins*Publishers*

Angus&Robertson

An imprint of HarperCollins*Publishers,* Australia

First published in Australia in 1996
Reprinted in 1996, 1997
by HarperCollins*Publishers* Pty Limited
ACN 009 913 517
A member of the HarperCollins*Publishers* (Australia) Pty Limited Group

HarperCollins*Publishers*
25 Ryde Road, Pymble, Sydney, NSW 2073, Australia
31 View Road, Glenfield, Auckland 10, New Zealand
77-85 Fulham Palace Road, London W6 8JB, United Kingdom
Hazelton Lanes, 55 Avenue Road, Suite 2900, Toronto, Ontario M5R 3L2
and 1995 Markham Road, Scarborough, Ontario M1B 5M8, Canada
10 East 53rd Street, New York NY 10032, USA

National Library of Australia Cataloguing-in-Publication data:

Horne, Ross.
Cancerproof your body.
Includes index.
ISBN 0 207 18900 5
1. Cancer–Nutritional aspects–Popular works. 2. Cancer–Prevention–Popular works.
3. Cancer–Diagnosis–Popular works. 4. Cancer–Diet therapy–Popular works. I. Title.
616.994052.

Printed in Australia by Griffin Press, Adelaide
9 8 7 6 5 4 3   97 98 99

Contents

'But nobody can say

that one does not know what

cancer and its prime cause can be.

On the contrary, there is no disease

whose prime cause is better known,

so that today ignorance is no excuse

that one cannot do more about prevention.

That prevention of cancer will come there is

no doubt, for man wishes to survive.

But how long prevention will be avoided

depends on how long the prophets of

agnosticism will succeed in inhibiting

the application of scientific knowledge

in the cancer field. In the meantime,

millions of men must

die of cancer unnecessarily.'

—Otto Warburg,
double Nobel Prize Laureate, 1966

Dedicated to the memory of
Robert Bell, MD

About the author and his work

by Dr Dean Burk,
former head of Cytochemistry Department,
US National Cancer Institute

Having spent most of my professional life in the field of cancer research — a field of great complexity and no little confusion — I was astonished and delighted to become acquainted with Ross Horne's book *The Health Revolution*.

My astonishment arises from the discovery that a layman (the author is a retired airline captain) should have gained such a comprehensive understanding of the complex biological processes which lead to the disease called 'cancer' and to be able to describe these processes in a manner easily understandable by other laymen. The author describes the origins of not only cancer but of other so-called diseases of civilisation and the natural measures required to avoid and control them.

When it is considered that few medical professionals possess this knowledge, this is no mean achievement.

The strength, integrity and happiness of a nation are directly proportional to the state of health of its citizens. In the distant past civilisations have risen, flourished and declined, their ruins covered by desert sands. Did affluence destroy them? Are we heading the same way?

Perhaps humans are too clever for their own good. In the pursuit of progress and pleasure they at the same time sow the seeds of their own destruction.

Modern man must comprehend the message presented in this book that the greatest threat to his survival is not that of nuclear war, because although that threat is real, at least everyone is aware of it. The threat most dangerous to mankind comes from the destroyers active right now, subtle and unseen — the poisoning of our soil and water supplies, the de-naturing of our food, the ever-increasing destruction of the environment.

No more do people die of old age; instead, heart attacks, strokes, cancer, diabetes and so on are today accepted as normal causes of death. Influenza, arthritis, indigestion, constipation, aches and pains and medicine are a normal part of life. Are coronary bypasses, hysterectomies, reading glasses, hearing aids, wheelchairs, false teeth and plastic hipjoints to be considered normal too?

On his long evolutionary journey, man has strayed on to dangerous ground. Now we are at a crossroads, and whichever way we take there will be some rough going. As ever, the fittest will survive.

Ross Horne's book is a survival manual for the trip ahead.

(This statement first appeared as the Foreword to Ross Horne's book, *The Health Revolution*. Dr Dean Burk (1904–88) was a foundation member of the US National Cancer Institute and former head of its Cytochemistry Department. He was best known for his work on cancer research for which he received honours from France, Britain, Germany and Russia. Formerly Associate Professor of Biochemistry, Cornell University, he worked in cancer research at the Kaiser Wilhelm Institute in Germany and at the Academy of Science in Moscow. Dr Burk received the Domagk Prize for cancer research, was a Knight Commander of the Medical Order of Bethlehem, and a Knight of the Mark Twain Society. He was co-author of the books *Cancer, Approaches to Tumour Chemotherapy* and *Cell Chemistry*, and author of over 250 published scientific papers.)

Introduction

'When a man's science exceedeth his sense,
he perishes by his ignorance.'
— Oriental proverb

In 1984 the Australian Broadcasting Corporation (ABC) produced a television program entitled *Understanding Cancer*, which presented the views of a number of eminent cancer specialists and research doctors. One by one the doctors, somewhat uncertainly, explained the subject of cancer as currently theorised in scientific circles, with the admission, both at the beginning and at the end of the program, that they didn't really understand cancer themselves. Since then nothing has changed — the bewilderment and confusion continues.

You would think that, after the intense research over many years at prodigious expense in the best equipped laboratories in the world, such research would have by now produced better than just another theory a theory that is highly scientific, but sadly lacking in commonsense in that it not only fails to accommodate many of the known facts, but conflicts with others. Surely in the mountains of research data that have accumulated the real key to explaining cancer must already exist.

The key in fact does exist — not only the key, but the complete explanation of the so-called mystery of cancer. But the medical profession, confused and led astray by one fashionable theory after another, has failed to comprehend the most fundamental fact: *all living things are governed by fixed and unchanging biological laws* that do not require space-age technology to interpret. Reference to these laws — laws laid down over billions of years of biological evolution — was the means by which a few more-discerning researchers of the past finally solved the mystery of cancer, but few people are aware of this.

The mystery solved, the problem that cancer now presents is in getting medical research out of the dead-end rut it has been in for so long and opening researchers' eyes to proven data they have overlooked. However, the long-suppressed facts are beginning to emerge; there is a glimmer of hope — doctors now talk, albeit hesitantly, about the protective role of green vegetables, something that natural-health practitioners have preached for over one hundred years. But there is a lot more for doctors to learn, and you cannot afford to wait for the 'experts' to catch up — it may take many more years.

The ABC program, despite its limitations, did provide some good advice based on its observation that an estimated 80% of all cancers were caused by environmental factors and thus were potentially preventable. This observation and its conclusion are only partly correct because, as the following chapters describe, *all cancers result from environmental factors and are therefore 100% preventable.*

The failure of modern 'scientific' medicine to solve the problem of cancer is due to the tenaciously held idea that cancer is a cellular aberration that can occur in an otherwise healthy body more due to bad luck than bad management, and that the cure for it is to cut it out or in some other way destroy it, a traumatic and expensive procedure that, as the statistics show, rarely succeeds (described in Appendix B).

The truth is that the irregular behaviour of cells in the body is a predictable result of a disordered condition of body chemistry and, when such irregular cells begin to grow as cancer, the resultant tumour is only a symptom of the deeper, more subtle disorder within.

The long-sought key to the cancer problem is to rectify the cause and not just to blindly attack the effect. Do not wait until the medical industry finally abandons the aspirations of discovering a cure for cancer (or for whatever else threatens), as diseases can only be cured if the causes of them are removed.

The object of this book is to acquaint the reader with a clear understanding of the following:

1. The easily avoidable processes within the body that lead to cancer

2. How cancer commences and grows

3. How, if the proper steps are taken, these processes can be reversed

It all gets back to proper management of the environment within your body — get this right, and not only can you avoid cancer but at the same time you can ensure you have complete freedom from all the other health problems that cause so much distress in the world today.

Ross Horne
January 1996

CHAPTER 1

The Hunzas

'Cancer is so rare [in the principality of Hunza] that in nine years practice I never came across a single case of it.'
—Major-General Sir Robert McCarrison,
British Army Medical Service

SHANGRI-LA

Shangri-la was an exquisitely beautiful valley somewhere among the great mountains of the Himalayas, a paradise on Earth, where people lived in perfect happiness. There was no crime in the valley, no sickness to mar the inhabitants' existence; the people of Shangri-la enjoyed perfect health and contentment.

Shangri-la was the setting for James Hilton's enchanting book, *Lost Horizon*, published in 1933. Movies have been made about it, and over the years there has always been speculation among romantics whether the legendary valley really existed.

Although Shangri-la exists only in the imagination of romantic people, there really does exist a valley high in the Himalayas which closely resembles it — the valley of Hunza. The valley lies at the foot of towering Mount Rakaposhi, where the Himalayas meet the Karakoram Range and the Hindu Kush, way up in the remote area where the boundaries of China, Tadzhikistan, Afghanistan and Pakistan all converge.

It is believed that the Hunza valley was the inspiration for James Hilton's book because over the past one hundred years or so the accounts given by various adventurers who have been there all glowingly praise the beauty and grandeur of the valley and the supreme health and splendid physique of its inhabitants.

Hunza was a tiny independant state until it became a part of Pakistan in 1947. Once isolated and inaccessible, in recent years Hunza has been made accessible by road, and no doubt this has brought about many changes.

A British doctor, Major-General Sir Robert McCarrison, who served many years in the British Army Indian Medical Service earlier this century, gave this account of his impressions of the Hunza people, as he encountered them in those days, living frugally but happily detached from the outside world:

> The power of endurance of these people is extraordinary: to see a man of this race throw off his scanty garments revealing a figure which would delight the eye of a Rodin, and plunge into a glacier-fed river in the middle of winter with as much unconcern as many of us would take a tepid bath, is to realise that perfection of physique and great physical endurance are attainable on the simplest of foods, providing these be of the right kind. These people are long-lived and vigorous in old age. Among the ailments so common in our own people — such as gastro-intestinal disorders, colitis, gastro and duodenal ulcer and cancer — are extraordinarily uncommon.
>
> With the Hunza, resistance to infection is remarkable ... gastro-intestinal complaints, dyspepsia, ulcers, colitis and appendicitis are at least as uncommon as they are common elsewhere. Cancer is so rare that in nine years practice I never came across a single case of it.

Upon his arrival in India as a young man, McCarrison, as Regimental Medical Officer, was responsible for the health of the Indian troops. He soon observed that the health and physical standards of the Indian population varied enormously from one region to another. The Hunzas, Pathans and Sikhs, McCarrison considered to be the finest specimens of humanity he had ever seen; on the other end of McCarrison's scale came the miserable, poorer classes of Bengal and Madras, among whom diseases of every description were common and life short.

He formed the opinion, after further investigation, that this great variation in health standards was the result of the difference in the sorts of food that formed the traditional diets in the different regions.

This opinion he proved correct in his famous dietary experiments with animals at Coonor in 1927. Using several thousand white rats caged in hygienic conditions, different groups of rats were selectively fed the different diets of various Indian regions. The results of the experiment were rapid and clear-cut: the animals fed on the Hunza diet displayed the physical excellence of the Hunza people — sleek, bright eyed, active and content — while the animals fed with the diet of the poor city-dwellers displayed all the appalling diseases so common to those people. Likewise, other rats fed the typical diet of the poor English classes of the time — white bread, margarine, boiled vegetables, tinned meats, and so on — soon displayed the bad health and stunted growth common among the English poor.

That is what a lawyer would call an 'open-and-shut case'. On the one hand you have a diet that in humans or in rats produces fine physique and perfect health, and on the other hand you have a diet than in humans or in rats brings about every disease known to humanity — including cancer. And what applied in 1927 applies equally today. Notwithstanding that since 1927 lots of additional health-threatening factors have been introduced into our environment, the main factor determining an individual's health and physique is still the sort of food eaten by that individual.

In 1927 only well-to-do people could afford the sort of food high in protein and fat that made them portly and gave them gout, but today most people in Western industrialised society can afford what is now known as 'the traditional Western diet', so that the poorer classes no longer die like flies from pneumonia and tuberculosis but instead live a few years longer to die of heart attacks and cancer just like wealthy people do. And the fact that heart specialists perish just as readily as everyone else from these maladies demonstrates pretty clearly that these people don't know nearly as much about their specialties as they should.

Therefore it can be seen that the status quo today is not that much better than in 1927, and in regard to cancer it is in fact a great deal worse. In 1927 cancer was responsible for only one death in about ten, whereas today it kills one person in four, and it is predicted that it will kill one in three people before the year 2000. These numbers are statistics, and you don't want to be one of them; you don't have to be, because you can make your body cancerproof.

Everyone today is aware of the importance of preserving the environment. The future welfare of humanity depends on it. However there is another environment which for your individual immediate welfare is more important still, and that is the environment existing within your own body. You should properly care for this environment within. If you do, you will not get cancer.

CHAPTER 2

Healthy blood, healthy cells, healthy body

'In Nature there are neither rewards or punishments ... there are consequences.' — Robert Ingersoll

Everyone knows that the body is made up of living cells, billions and billions of them, but few people stop to consider that each and every cell of which they are made is, in its own right, an individual living organism. Each cell in fact is a citizen, as it were, of a tightknit community of cells. The cell's first concern of course is its own survival, its second concern being its contribution to the best interests of its community of fellow cells.

If each and every cell of the body is well-nourished and healthy, then so too will the whole body be healthy.

CELLS

Examined under a microscope, the cells of the different body tissues are dissimilar and can be identified as to what kind they are — for example, lung-tissue cells, skin cells, or bone cells — because they vary in size and structure according to their function.

Different as they may be, it is an incredible fact that every one of them is a descendant of one parent cell: the fertilised egg cell, which shortly after conception sub-divides into two cells, again into four, and so on. In this very early stage of pregnancy the cells all look alike — they are 'undifferentiated' — and multiply rapidly as if out of control. As the embryo grows, the cells change into different forms and groups — the process of differentiation — and so begins the construction of the different organs of the body. As this process continues, each new generation of cells becomes more and more different and specialised, while at the same time the cells' multiplication becomes 'controlled' and slows down, until the body is complete, at which stage the cells are said to be fully differentiated.

It is interesting to note that just after conception the undifferentiated embryo cells resemble primitive single-cell life forms still to be found in the sea, which reflects the fact that it was from such primitive organisms that the higher forms of life evolved. Further demonstrating this evolutionary process is the fact that in the early stages of development the human embryo resembles almost exactly the embryos of all the other animals on Earth, even at one stage having gills like a fish, and later, a tail, features which disappear as differentiation proceeds.

These interesting facts about evolution and cell differentiation are described here because some understanding of them enables us to accept that the complex and mysterious processes that take place within our bodies all the time are governed by fixed, long established laws of Nature, and that all diseases — including cancer — are direct biological consequences of departures from these laws.

THE ENVIRONMENT WITHIN

To achieve a state in which the various completed organs of the human body function as they are meant to, all the while protected by a fully functional immune system, the environment within the body must be kept just right.

The principle of total body health being directly related to the purity of the fluid environment in which the body cells dwell was conceived by the great French physiologist Professor Claude Bernard in the 19th century. Bernard coined the term *milieu interieur*, which means 'environment within'.

This gently flowing fluid is called 'lymph', or 'interstitial fluid', and consists of plasma — the clear liquid component of the blood — which seeps from the capillary vessels of the main blood circulation into the body tissues to deliver oxygen and nutrients to the cells and to convey cells' waste products away for elimination. The 'spent' lymph returns to the main blood circulation by way of the lymphatic system — a separate network of blood vessels, similar to veins — and is propelled by the squeezing action that occurs with muscle movements of ordinary activity, and better still by exercise of a more vigorous kind.

(It is an interesting fact that the chemical composition of lymph is almost the same as seawater, which again reflects the fact that the cells of our bodies are descendants of the first single-celled sea creatures that preceded the higher forms of life billions of years ago.)

The purity of the lymph surrounding each cell obviously depends on the quality of the blood and the vigour of the circulation, the cleansing action of the lymph being as important as the nourishing action. And, in turn, the quality of the blood is dependent primarily on the efficiency of the liver and kidneys and, ahead of that, on the quality of the food and water from which the body makes new blood.

When the quality of the *milieu interieur* is just right, the blood and lymph flow freely, rich in nutrients and oxygen and free of unwanted substances or toxins; the oxygen-carrying red cells of the blood float freely and so too do

THE EYE OF THE HUNZA
by Allen E Banik

One of my major reasons for wanting to visit Hunza was to find out whether their robust health would be corroborated by evidence of superior circulatory function as revealed by a study of the arteries and veins within their eyes, also to learn if their eyesight was superior, in general, to that of our population.

Although optometrists do not practise medicine, their knowledge of pathology enables them to refer patients with abnormalities to proper medical authority.In my opinion, comparison of the diameters of the arteries and veins of the eye indicates whether the circulatory system is 'in balance' or 'out of balance' — whether a person's blood pressure is normal or abnormal. Determination of the colour relationship between arteries and veins is also indicative of an individual's condition. For example, if the colour ratio between an artery and corresponding vein is 1:1, a person is healthy (i.e. the artery is rich red and the vein has a colour intensity of equal degree). If the colour ratio is 1:2 (the vein is two shades darker than the artery), health is somewhat below normal. The average American — including many children — falls into this category. A ratio of 1:3 indicates illness: at approaching death the ratio is 1:4.

Interesting evidence of this theory is supplied by studies made by Dr Melvin Knisely of the University of Chicago. Dr Knisely made an exhaustive study of the colour changes in the circulatory systems of dying frogs, monkeys and humans, and was able to predict the progression of diseases. As death approached, the toxin-laden corpuscles were unable to pass through the capillaries. Their progress was stopped and their oxygen content discharged. As a sticky substance in the blood covered the dying cells they formed into clusters which the doctor called 'blood sludge' — a condition common in fifty diseases. Gradually, the blood flowed more slowly, and the tissues died of asphyxia. 'Understanding sludge,' Dr Knisely says, 'will make possible a new attack on a whole panorama of human diseases.' Photomicrographs of the circulatory systems of frogs, monkeys and humans substantiated the theory. An account of this remarkable discovery appeared in Life magazine, 31 May 1948.

The examinations I made in Hunza of the eyes of people in all age groups indicated that the Hunzakuts have healthy circulatory systems. Their artery-to-vein circumference ratios were, in most cases, perfect or near perfect, and the colour ratios could generally be classified at 1:1.

In all respects the Hunzakuts' eyes were notable. I found them unusually clear; there were few signs of astigmatism; even the oldest men had excellent far and near vision — an indication that their crystalline lenses had retained elasticity. Most of our crystalline lenses lose their elasticity in our early forties, and we require bifocal lenses for the remainder of our lives.

Here, I believe, is confirmation of the fact that bodily health can be 'read' by a study of the eyes, and that general health promotes eye health. For our own benefit and that of our children, we should resolve that, starting now, we will make the necessary adjustments in our diet to promote the radiant health to which we are all entitled.

Source: Allen E Banik, *Hunza Land*, Whitehorn Publishing Co, Long Beach, California, 1960.

the protective white cells of the immune system, vigorous and efficient. When this ideal condition is achieved, all the organs of the body harmonise and everything works the way it should. The condition of perfectly balanced body chemistry is called 'homeostasis', a term popularised by another great physiologist, Walter Cannon, MD ScD, of Harvard University. In his classic book, *The Wisdom of the Body*, Dr Cannon explained how, regardless of conditions that varied widely, the 'body wisdom' works constantly to maintain homeostasis.

If there are any deficiencies in nutrition, if there exists any form of toxaemia or if there is inadequate oxygen or poor circulation or organ malfunction, the body will attempt to maintain homeostasis, but if it cannot, the *milieu interieur* will suffer, and with it the health of the cells and the whole body. The way the body reacts will depend upon the extent and manner in which homeostasis is upset. One way or another, the body will be ill at ease — in other words, dis-eased — and so, according to whatever symptoms the body displays, one or another of a textbook-full of medical names will be given to these symptoms.

The most troublesome of the factors commonly degrading the *milieu interieur* are various forms of toxaemia and various nutritional deficiencies, both factors being consequences of improper diet. In most cases the diet is reasonably adequate in necessary nutrients, but the problem of malnutrition nevertheless exists because of:

1. Excesses of some dietary components, the worst being fat and protein (mainly from meat and dairy products), and excessive amounts of grain products
2. The denaturing effect of cooking
3. The inclusion of harmful substances, such as salt, condiments and refined sugar

Thus everybody enjoying our time-honoured traditional foods — home-cooked or (worse still) take-away — is rendered prone to health problems, minor enough in youth but worsening with age.

As toxaemia can occur in countless different forms and degrees — not only through improper diet but also through stress, absence of fresh air and sunshine, lack of exercise, smoking, and taking alcohol, drugs and medicine — once the limits of 'body wisdom' are exceeded, the resultant effects may vary widely. This explains why there are so many diseases listed in medical textbooks and why doctors, not realising the true nature of the problem, go to so much trouble to decide which 'disease' is 'attacking' the patient when all the time nothing is attacking the patient at all. Explained at the same time are why there are so many diseases of 'unknown aetiology' (that is, of unknown cause or origin) and why so many people suffer and die from medical treatment aimed at the symptom while ignoring the real disease, which is the absence of homeostasis.

When the usual blood tests are made for chronically sick people, the blood is assessed for various chemical elements and compounds, and a count is made of the red blood cells (erythrocytes) and white blood cells (leucocytes). A more thorough inspection of the blood under a microscope, however, reveals a lot more.

In all conditions of chronic disease the blood is shown to be polluted with sludge. The term 'blood sludge' was coined by Dr Melvin H Knisely of the University of Chicago and the Medical College of South Carolina, and is used to describe the pathological blood condition technically known as 'intravascular erythrocyte aggregation'. This condition, first described in medical literature in 1754 by Dr A Haller of London as 'a concreted tremulous jelly throughout all the veins', has been recognised by many other doctors since then in all chronic conditions of disease. Blood sludge is also called 'intravascular agglutination of the blood', 'red cell agglutination', 'blood cell agglutination' and 'granular flow'.

In all conditions of chronic disease the blood is seen to be sticky (of high viscosity), and the red cells and blood platelets tend to stick together (that is, aggregate) so that the blood cannot carry oxygen properly and it cannot circulate properly.

In addition, as the blood pollution worsens, various virus-like microorganisms make their appearance and are frequently mistaken to be the cause of the inevitable pathological conditions that develop.

This condition, of course, is a demonstration of a diseased *milieu interieur*, reflected in medical tests by high blood pressure, high erythrocyte sedimentation rate (ESR) and a high score on the platelet adhesion index (PAI). Briefly, the ESR is the rate at which red cells settle to the bottom of the blood sample: the higher the rate, the worse the condition of the blood. The red cells sink faster, despite the increased stickiness of the blood plasma in which they float, because in clumps they are denser than free-floating cells. The PAI is an index that measures the stickiness of blood platelets.

As blood sludge is caused mainly by excess fat and protein in the diet, it can be cleared in a few days by strict dietary correction or, even better, by fasting. The improvement in wellbeing is rapid and startling.

Although it is common knowledge among doctors that these poor blood conditions accompany the various chronic problems they are trying to treat, the reason they do not succeed in restoring their patients to health is that their orthodox training does not permit them to see that the impure, sticky, sludged blood is not just an accompaniment of the patient's complaint — in most cases it is the *cause* of the patient's complaint.

Thus medical drugs can, at best, do no more than dull or remove the symptoms; in the long run they can do nothing but harm to the patient because, being substances unnatural to the body, they place further strain on the already overworked organs, which correctly sense a drug to be a toxic substance to be neutralised and expelled. In this way medical drugs, many of which have been shown to be quite dangerous, are counterproductive to the integrity of the *milieu interieur* and cause additional distress casually referred to as 'side effects', the worst side of which, all too often, is death.

Animals in their natural environment are sleek and healthy all through their lives, while most modern-day humans are rarely sleek and too often have something wrong with them until finally despatched, usually by heart disease, stroke or cancer. The 'diseases of civilisation' don't happen to animals in the wild whose bodies are no better designed than ours.

Do animals know something that humans don't know? The answer is no. To the contrary, humans know something that animals do not: we know how to take natural food and make it unnatural, we even know how to take unnatural food and make is more unnatural, all the while making it delightful to eat — without, however, realising that it strains our digestive organs and pollutes our blood. We know how to flavour food with salt and condiments, and how to wash it all down with wine, beer, coffee and tea.

In short, we have elevated the practice of eating to an intensely pleasurable art form in which eating is encouraged as much by a craving for addictive tastes, such as sugar and salt, as it is by genuine hunger, so leading to the over-indulgence that overloads our vital organs, pollutes our blood, and diminishes our vitality. Our cells get sick and we get sick.

CHAPTER 3

What is cancer?

'Struggling against cancer means not just fighting an occasional enemy who strikes at random and unjustly. It means learning little by little to master the very conditions of life, its maintenance and equilibrium at the level of the cell and at the level of the great overall regulatory mechanisms.'
— Lucien Israel, MD, Head of Hospital Franco, Musulman, Bobigney, France

Various tissues make up the structure of all living things, and these tissues are composed of countless numbers of tiny cells, each cell with a life of its own but at all times living and cooperating in perfect harmony with all of the other cells, as long as healthy conditions exist.

The lifespan of an individual cell in the human body is brief. As cells wear out — which millions of them do every minute — they are replaced by new ones, produced by healthy cells dividing into two. Apart from this constant replacement of cells through normal wear-and-tear, in a similar fashion new cells are made when necessary to heal tissue that has been injured in any way.

In a healthy body these processes occur rapidly and in a strictly controlled way, so that only the required numbers of new cells are made and no more. These constraints to growth exist in all tissues of the body and are automatic and unfailing, as long as the tissues are in a sound and healthy condition.

But sometimes, due to influences not yet understood within the medical profession, one or more cells somewhere in the body begin to behave abnormally and, in defiance of the existing constraints, commence to reproduce needlessly. Should this abnormal reproduction of faulty cells continue, the resultant growth is cancer: called in medical terms a 'tumour' or 'neoplasm'.

Whereas it is commonly assumed that cancer can arise within normal tissue in a healthy body, it will no doubt already be apparent to the reader that this cannot happen. Cancer never occurs in healthy tissue that is well nourished and has good circulation. It is now becoming recognised in medical circles that cancer is usually a gradual process in a slowly degenerating body.

THE CANCER PROCESS

The term 'pre-cancer' is used to describe the unhealthy condition of tissue which always precedes cancer — a condition of imperfect body chemistry known as the 'cancer milieu', which is often reflected by various constitutional disorders, vague ill health and fatigue. In the view of some researchers, cancer begins with the initial degeneration of the tissues, but most consider it to start with the beginning of the first tumour, which is the first undeniable evidence of its existence. *One way or the other, the only solution to the problem of cancer is to clean up the cancer milieu that underlies this disease as well as underlying many others.*

Cancer, in the location where it first starts, is called a 'primary cancer' or a 'primary tumour'. Primary cancer most commonly occurs in the epithelial tissues (the tissues of the skin and of the membranes), as these are the tissues in which the normal renewal of cells is greatest.

Epithelial tissues include the lining of the digestive tract, respiratory tract, kidneys, the female genital tract and, of course, the 'outside' skin. Cancers in epithelial tissues are called 'carcinomas' and account for 90% of all human cancer deaths.

Primary tumours occur less frequently in connective tissue and bones, which have a slower turnover of normal cells anyway. These tumours are called 'sarcomas'.

Cancer of the blood and blood-forming tissue is called 'leukemia', and in lymphatic tissue it is called 'lymphoma'. Primary cancer never occurs in nerve tissues, which are tissues in which the changeover of cells does not occur.

The degree of malignancy of a cancer depends on the degree to which the cells in it have become abnormal. Cells which are only slightly abnormal differ only slightly in appearance to the normal cells of their origin, and can be easily identified as being lung cells or kidney cells or whatever, and they still partially respond to the normal restraints to growth. Thus a slow-growing self-contained tumour may be considered benign and to be presenting no immediate danger.

The most malignant cancers are those composed of cells that have become so abnormal they can hardly be identified at all, and which respond even less to attempted restraints to growth and so grow faster. At the same time, malignant cancers liberate stray cancer cells capable of travelling in the body fluids to other locations.

Most of these travelling cancer cells are intercepted by the defensive white cells of the immune system and are destroyed, but as people with cancer generally have depressed immune systems, cancer cells often escape and, if one should lodge in a clogged-up blood vessel or some other 'safe spot' long enough to gain a foothold, it may continue to reproduce to form a new tumour, called a 'secondary tumour'.

Although in a different location in the body, a secondary tumour when it starts is made up of cells still the same as those of the primary tumour. Thus when cancer is first discovered, identification will tell whether it is a primary tumour on its home ground or a secondary tumour from some other site. For instance, a tumour in the lung may be a primary made of cancerous lung cells or turn out to be a secondary made of cancerous kidney cells. Often there are multiple secondaries.

When secondary cancer starts, the cancer is said to be 'metastasised'. Metastasised cancer is more dangerous than primary cancer because the automatic constraints to growth, although present in all parts of the body, differ from one location to another and are effective only in controlling cells situated in their normal tissue of origin. This means that, in a different location, the cells of a secondary tumour are no longer restrained at all and are free to multiply as they wish.

If no measures are taken to arrest the course of cancer, death will be the eventual outcome. In some cases the cancer growth may obstruct some vital body function, sometimes it destroys a blood vessel to cause a fatal haemorrhage. Sometimes the body becomes so depleted that, in the absence of immune system resistance, some infection takes over. More often than not death occurs in the condition of cachexia, which is where the cancer cells have robbed the body of nutritional sustenance and poisoned it with their accumulated toxic waste products.

In brief, the unrestrained growth of cancer is a vicious circle: the cancer continually worsens the conditions that started it off in the first place, while at the same time wastefully consuming more and more of the body's limited nourishment and converting it to poisonous waste beyond the body's capacity to excrete.

Summarising, cancer is a procession of stages:

Stage 1 Pre-cancer, a condition of imperfect body chemistry.

Stage 2 The advent of primary cancer.

Stage 3 The progression of primary cancer.

Stage 4 Metastasis, the advent of secondary cancer.

Stage 5 Cachexia.

THE ORTHODOX VIEWPOINT

An indication of how little the medical professionals understand the subject of cancer, and why, as a result, they have such little success in treating the disease, can be seen in the way the stages of cancer are medically categorised:

Stage 1 Primary cancer, established but confined to its location of origin.

Stage 2 Evidence of spread to local lymph nodes but still regionally confined.

Stage 3 Extensive primary cancer and extensive involvement of the lymph nodes.

Stage 4 Metastasised cancer.

From this medical classification it can be seen that the orthodox medical viewpoint of cancer focuses only on the growth itself, and totally ignores the fact that a pre-cancerous state of the body's entire constitution must exist, possibly for many years, before primary cancer makes its first appearance.

To emphasise this medical shortcoming, the conventional advice in regard to warning signs of cancer is woefully inadequate. The seven 'warning signs' formulated by the American Cancer Society are:

1. Change in bowel or bladder habits.

2. A sore that does not heal.

3. Unusual bleeding or discharge.

4. Thickening or lump under the skin anywhere.

5. Indigestion or difficulty in swallowing.

6. Obvious change in a wart or mole.

7. Nagging cough or hoarseness.

These warning signs are valid enough but are not early warnings: they are indications of established cancer, already probably quite advanced, and possibly already metastasised.

EARLY SIGNS

Preceding the actual symptoms of advanced cancer, there are however many earlier signs of cancer or pre-cancer to provide advance warning. Cancer specialist and researcher Dr Cornelius Moerman of Holland lists these early signs as follows:

• Dry, cracked, scaly or horny skin

• Changes in mucous membranes

• Unhealthy colour of tongue and inside lips

• Rhagades (chaps or fissures of the skin) at corner of mouth

• Scaly rings around nose

• Nails hard and crumbly with line formations

- Hair dry and dead looking
- Signs of oedema on inside lower leg
- Low vitality (accompanied with lower than normal temperature)
- Bleeding gums
- Easy bruising
- Slow healing of wounds
- Symptoms of anaemia, alkalosis, poor blood
- Poor appetite, loss of weight
- The appearance and multiplication in the blood of virus-like microorganisms

Taken singly these signs are not necessarily indications of cancer, Dr Moerman said, but in combination they are.

In Chapter 5 reference is made to the now generally discarded virus theory of cancer based on the suspicion that a virus form of organism commonly discerned in the blood of cancer patients was the probable cause of the cancer. Dr Guy Owens, a surgeon in Amarillo, Texas, believes, like Dr Moerman, that the virus is a sign but not the cause; that is, this virus indicates a pre-cancerous condition that will eventually lead to cancer. He said in 1979:

> We selected 25 cases from my practice where the organisms were repeatedly found during blood counts. They were run of the mill office cases, being male, female, old and young, but apparently in average good health. Over a 20 year period, 23 of these people came down with malignancy of one kind or another ... proven by surgery and proper pathological examination. Two cases were lost from our records although one was known to have died from an obscure abdominal condition.

Dr Robert Bell, in his book *The Cancer Scourge*, noted that cancer was usually, but not invariably, preceded by other symptoms of deterioration — which included rheumatism, constipation, languor, dyspepsia and ovarian disease — all of which were accompanied and brought about by an unhealthy blood condition. Dr Bell considered the most accurate predictor of all of these problems was the condition of the blood as determined by visual, microscopic examination of a blood sample.

All degenerative conditions must be considered as indicative of a deteriorated state of the body's entire constitution which, when sufficiently deteriorated, becomes the cancer milieu.

There is a tendency for doctors to regard cancers appearing in different organs of the body as being different diseases, and to study each one separately, and to prepare statistics accordingly. When the statistics are compared, however, they merely demonstrate that cancer is the same disease occurring in different places.

It is the cancer milieu that is the real disease, and cancer is the major and final symptom of it.

REMEMBER

Clearing the cancer milieu and restoring a sound constitution can be accomplished in most cases simply by strict dietary correction, but is more effectively accomplished by combining dietary correction with a program of stress removal, light exercise, and exposure to fresh air and sunshine. In many cases such a program can bring about a remission of even well-established cancer, an event known as spontaneous remission.

SKIN 'CANCERS'

The lesions of the skin that are commonly called skin 'cancers' are, in most cases, not cancers at all: they are the scabs of skin tissue that has not developed properly, usually due to prior injury of sub-surface immature skin cells by the sun.

We are constantly warned by medical authorities that sunlight is the dangerous factor, but two additional factors must be borne in mind:

1. Now that more people are becoming diet-conscious and switching to low fat diets, they notice that they no longer get skin 'cancers', regardless of sun exposure.

2. Similar skin lesions frequently occur on skin seldom exposed to the sun anyway.

Keratoacanthoma is a more pronounced form of benign growth. It occurs in the skin and is also due to injury to immature sub-surface skin cells before they reach the surface. Upon their arrival at the surface these cells fail to differentiate properly, and form a growth that gradually extends in area and may be mistaken for a real carcinoma. However, it extends no further than the area affected. If the tissue is otherwise healthy the abnormal cells eventually die, a scab forms, and the skin returns to normal.

In one case known to myself, a keratoacanthoma, about 25 millimetres (1 inch) in diameter, occurred on the forearm of a writer who used a strong spotlight positioned behind his right shoulder. The spotlight was so powerful it discoloured the fabric of the chair's armrest. In the usual course of events the growth would have been removed surgically, but this treatment was refused. After several weeks the lump turned into a scab, which simply fell off and left just a trace of a scar. Whether such a lesion could lead to a real carcinoma would be dependent on whether or not a pre-cancerous condition existed in the first place. In healthy tissue cancer cannot exist.

CHAPTER 4

Who gets cancer and who doesn't?

'It is abundantly clear that the incidence of all the common cancers in humans is being determined by various potentially controllable external factors, because people in different parts of the world suffer from different kinds of cancer, depending on their habits, diet and customs rather than on their ethnic origins. Thus, when people migrate from one country to another they tend to acquire the pattern of cancer that is characteristic of their new home. This is surely the most comforting fact to come out of all cancer research, for it means cancer is, in large part, a preventable disease.' — National Research Council, USA, Diet, Nutrition and Cancer

Epidemiology is the study of the occurrence, transmission and control of disease in different population groups. The many epidemiological studies conducted over the last hundred years or so clearly indicate that human cancers of all kinds are the result of lifestyle errors that, in one way or another, compromise the purity of the body's internal fluids, blood and lymph, because (as already explained in Chapter 2) it is the condition of these fluids that determines the health status of each and every one of the countless cells out of which the body is made. The lymph (interstitial fluid) — which bathes the cells and provides them with nutrients and oxygen, as well as cleansing them of their waste products — is derived directly from the main bloodstream, and so it is self-evident that no part of the body can function properly unless the bloodstream is pure and free-flowing.

THE DIET CONNECTION

Of all the errors possible in day-to-day living, the one that more than any other compromises the integrity of the bloodstream is imperfect nutrition.

FOOD AND YOU

From the moment you were conceived, when you consisted of only one single cell, right up until you were born, and further through childhood to adulthood (at which stage your body is now made of trillions of cells), every part of you — skin, blood, bones, muscles, down to your toenails — is made from substances derived from food. Not only are the right substances required for the body's growth and maintenance, but also for the making of the complicated hormones, vitamins and enzymes upon which the different intricate life processes depend. Suitable nutrients are also required to provide fuel for energy.

The more suitable the food is, the more trouble-free and efficient will the body be; conversely, the more unsuitable the food is, the more likely it is that the body's physique will suffer and disease be encountered.

Suitable food provides all the body's nutritional requirements in *natural* form. It allows the normal processes of digestion, general metabolism and elimination to proceed with minimum effort and without the production of toxic by-products capable of compromising the purity of the blood.

HOMEOSTASIS

When ideal conditions exist within the body, the body is said to be in chemical balance: not only will the blood chemistry be right, but the blood viscosity will be low, allowing the blood to be free-flowing and fully loaded with oxygen. When this has been achieved the body is said to be in a condition of homeostasis, a condition in which disease cannot occur.

Homeostasis is relatively easy to maintain when young — even on a diet that is mediocre or includes junk food, soft drinks and liquor — because the vital organs of digestion, purification and elimination, although suffering overwork, can still cope. But, as we age, our organs' capacity to cope diminishes with wear and tear: homeostasis will be progressively lost, and various symptoms of body malfunction will be increasingly displayed.

Depending on the manner in which any number of dietary factors may be involved in the disturbance of homeostasis, one or more different symptoms may be displayed, each one of which to the medically trained mind represents a different disease with its own classification and name. A condition or disease might be labelled asthma, arthritis, hypertension, diabetes, cataract, glaucoma, prostatitis, multiple sclerosis, osteoporosis, kidney failure, or heart disease — but it will represent in fact nothing more than a disruption of homeostasis. Cancer in its early stages fits the same pattern and, like the others, is easily reversible if proper measures are taken to restore homeostasis. However, if proper measures are *not* taken, the degree of malignancy will increase in a vicious circle, because the cancer increasingly contributes to the toxic milieu that brought it about in the first place.

Although it is known that many external environmental factors (including stress) are capable of degrading the body's chemical balance and thus contribute to the potential for cancer, and while such factors may cause irritation or damage to tissue, they have never been shown to be capable of directly causing cancer (that is, of changing normal tissue cells into cancer cells).

Whenever such irritation or tissue damage eventuates in cancer it only does so as a precipitative influence when a pre-cancerous condition already exists and, whenever this is the case, the evidence shows that improper diet is almost invariably the major factor in producing pre-cancer. It could hardly be otherwise: cancer happens to teetotallers as well as to drinkers, to non-smokers as well as to smokers, to farm workers as well as to city workers, and so on, and while such various lifestyle factors certainly influence a person's chances of developing cancer, they don't influence them as much as what is taken into the body three times a day or more, day in, day out, directly into the bloodstream by way of the stomach.

A DISEASE OF DEGENERATION

Major-General McCarrison reported that, in Hunza, cancer was unknown, and in other underdeveloped countries, cancer is extremely rare. The highest incidence of cancer (and the highest incidence of all the other degenerative diseases) occurs in the most affluent 'developed' countries, which are 'blessed' with bountiful quantities of meat, chicken, dairy products, fast foods and processed, canned and packaged foods — the sort of food commonly called 'the Western diet'.

We are led to believe the Western diet, which is supposedly 'balanced' by the inclusion of cooked grain products and a minor quantity of vegetables and fruit, makes us the best-fed people in the world. If 'best-fed' means overweight, constipated, and addicted to rich spicy food, then maybe we are the best-fed. But if we take into account the fact that we display the world's highest rates of coronary heart disease, stroke, cancer, asthma, diabetes, arthritis and so on, then it would be closer to the truth to say that we, supposedly civilised and progressive people, may be the worst fed.

The best epidemiological studies of cancer were recorded in the years before the ways of the white man became adopted in what were once regarded as the 'primitive' parts of the world. In 1927 Dr E H Tipper of England wrote a book called *The Cradle of the World and Cancer*, in which he said:

Cancer has been suspected of being a disease of civilisation. Judging by my experience in general practice in London, twenty years in West Africa, and again in rural England, I am convinced that this is true. It is due to the conventionalism and bad feeding of civilisation, and is an exact index of the degree to which the alimentary tract has deviated from its natural and normal state of health.

And in further reference to the African tribespeople and their simple diet he added: 'There is no such thing as constipation and there is no cancer. At the first dawn of civilisation amongst them, the disease makes its appearance; where civilisation is advanced, it is rife.'

The same thing has happened to the American Indians, Hawaiians, the Maoris, New Guineans and the Australian Aboriginies. Most recently, it has happened to the Nauruans, whose new-found wealth from their phosphate bounties enables them to live in comparative luxury but with escalating rates of diabetes, heart disease, cancer and the rest of the white man's physical problems.

However, there are still various population groups subsisting on their traditional simple diets who remain for the most part free of the so-called 'diseases of civilisation'. For instance, in the rural areas of Thailand and Vietnam heart disease and cancer are rare and it is an interesting fact that, after the Vietnam War, when American POWs were repatriated back to the USA, it was the first time in history that liberated POWs were in better physical health than when taken prisoner — a situation brought about by their involuntary abstinence from American food.

A similar comparison has been made between population groups within the USA, showing that you don't need to be a POW in Vietnam to reduce your risk of cancer and heart disease. Noted American cardiologist Jeremiah Stamler, MD, reporting on a study conducted by the Loma Linda University, explains:

> An additional comparison has recently become available, with data on mortality, for three groups of Californian Seventh Day Adventists — non vegetarian, lacto-ovo vegetarian [those who eat eggs and dairy foods] and pure vegetarian — compared with the Californian general population. Seventh Day Adventists have lower mean cholesterol levels than Americans generally. For 47,000 Seventh Day Adventist men aged 35 and over, age–sex-standardised, mortality rates were 34% lower for non vegetarians, 57% lower for the lacto-ovo vegetarians and 77% lower for the pure vegetarians compared with the general population. Seventh Day Adventists differ from the general population in other respects as well, e.g. abstinence from both alcohol and tobacco.

That different dietary faults are capable of producing different symptoms of disease, including different types of cancer, is illustrated by comparisons between the Japanese, the Americans, and Japanese who have migrated to America. The Japanese on their traditional, low fat, highly salted diet based on cooked rice and cooked vegetables with very little fruit have always displayed a high incidence of stomach cancer and a low incidence of colon cancer, whereas Americans on their traditional Western diet high in cooked animal protein, fat and sugar display a low incidence of stomach cancer and a high incidence of colon cancer. When Japanese migrate to the USA and settle in to American ways and eating habits they, as you might expect, soon lose their susceptibility to stomach cancer and increase their susceptibility to colon cancer.

The same trend has been observed in recent years in Japan itself, as the Western lifestyle becomes more and more popular there. As the Japanese consume more vegetables and fruit, their incidence of stomach cancer decreases; as they consume more and more meat and fat, their incidence of bowel cancer increases.

THE COOKED DIET

Humans world-wide are dependent to a great extent on cooked foods — especially grain products and meat, which are not ideal foods for human nutrition (and, in the case of grains, indigestible unless cooked).

The universal practice of cooking food changes its molecular structure, and while making it generally more palatable and easier to eat, it depletes the food's nutritional value and tends to destroy nutritional components, vitamins and natural enzymes protective against cancer. Worse still, it can produces chemical changes — in meat, in particular — capable of actually causing cancer. It is inevitable, then, that even the people we consider to be the healthiest are not perfect.

(Domestic dogs and cats fed only on the best quality canned meat suffer all kinds of human-like diseases, such as arthritis and cancer, as they get older; fed on raw meat, they remain healthy and live much longer. To rejuvenate your dog or cat try feeding it raw meat only, and observe the result.)

THE PRITIKIN DIET

The late Nathan Pritikin used to claim that the Pritikin diet was the best diet in the world and that, apart from anything else, it was the world's best defence against bowel cancer because a high grain diet provided sufficient fibre to keep the bowel swept clean of dangerous bacteria.

I used to believe it was the best in the world, and a lot of Pritikin followers still do, but in 1988 I felt obliged to write another book, called *Improving on Pritikin*, because of my observations of various injurious effects caused by diets, like Pritikin's, which encourage a high usage of grain products. Arthritis was the most common problem, the first case coming to my notice being the return of arthritis in my own right elbow after 25 years of good riddance. But the real incentive to warn people about such diets was the occurrence of cancer among a number of those who were long-term adherents to the Pritikin diet containing large quantities of grain products. Pritikin himself was dying from lymphoma when he ended his life in 1985.

Until this time I had been puzzled by some of the findings of the US Multiple Risk Factor Intervention Trial (MRFIT). The aim of the trial was to ascertain the extent to which the risk of heart disease could be reduced by diet or drugs. The trial took six years and studied 12,000 males.

The results confirmed the relationship between high cholesterol levels and heart disease, but at the same time they revealed a puzzling relationship between low cholesterol levels and cancer. Of the 12,000 subjects, those with medium and high cholesterol levels throughout the trial experienced death rates from cancer which were about the same as each other; but the group achieving the lowest levels of serum cholesterol (below 4.3 mm per litre, or 168 mg), while showing only a quarter of the death rate from heart disease than the high group, surprisingly had a death rate from cancer 50% *greater*! Some people immediately jumped to the conclusion it was dangerous to get serum cholesterol levels so low — a conclusion that contradicts the fact that the populations of the world with the lowest cholesterol levels display the lowest incidence of cancer, as well as the lowest incidence of heart disease.

So, ruling out low cholesterol as a reason for the higher death rate from cancer of this group, there are other factors to be taken into account.

First, had the high cholesterol groups not lost so many people to heart problems, a fair number of these people would have died of cancer instead, which would tend to even up the numbers.

Secondly, as cholesterol-lowering drugs are ineffectual compared to a cholesterol-lowering diet, and as only diet has been demonstrated effective enough to lower serum cholesterol below 4.3 mm per litre (168 mg%), diet must have been the main factor responsible for the higher incidence of cancer.

As Nathan Pritikin had already demonstrated before the MRFIT trial began, the only way to achieve such big reductions in blood cholesterol is to eliminate almost entirely from the diet all cholesterol-containing foods and in their place substitute cholesterol-free foods such as grain products, lentils, vegetables and fruit. The Pritikin diet works wonderfully to lower cholesterol and to improve circulation, but because (a) too little fruit is eaten, and (b) vegetables are eaten mostly cooked and are not very satisfying, and (c) grain products and lentils are not limited and *are* satisfying, it is the grain products and lentils that are consumed in excessive quantities capable of producing acid toxaemia, despite the fact constipation may no longer exist.

During the period of the trial, the Pritikin diet and the Macrobiotic diet were the only diets well known to be so effective in reducing cholesterol.

Both these diets are very high in grain products. Whatever benefit the fibre conveyed by keeping the bowel swept clean of dangerous bacteria, it would have been outweighed by the chemical imbalance caused by excessive acid production from eating so much grains and grain products. In the case of the Pritikin devotees mentioned before, none of them were on cholesterol-lowering drugs.

Grains contain much starch, which is not a good form of food: it is incomplete and at the same time difficult to digest, overtaxing the pancreas. Wheat is full of starch and contains gluten and phytic acid, which are also antagonistic to good body chemistry.

Studies of population groups in areas of Iran where the people are dependent mainly on wheat for food, show exceptionally high rates of cancer of the oesophagus.

In Africa the Bantu people, who rely mainly on corn for food, have an extremely high incidence of liver cancer although it is believed these people suffer some poisoning of the liver from the iron entering their food from the iron pots in which the food is traditionally cooked. Animal studies have confirmed, however, the corn meal diet to be responsible. (Max Gerson discusses this in *A Cancer Therapy: Results of Fifty Cases*.)

Possibly the strongest association of dietary faults with cancer is revealed in Dr Neils Dungal's observations, over a 40-year period, of the Icelanders. During this period the population was mainly dependent on a diet composed of smoked or salted meat, smoked or salted fish, animal fats, some dairy products and cereal, with no fruit or vegetables other than potatoes. During this period he found that stomach cancer was rare among fishermen but frequent among farmers, and that the Icelandic population exhibited the highest rate of stomach cancer in the world, with high rates of other cancers as well. Dr Dungal observed, in experiments with laboratory rats, it was the smoked meat and fish that produced the most stomach cancer.

There is strong medical support for the belief that many cancers might be prevented by eliminating chemical irritants from food. Malignant growths of the human digestive tract tend to appear in the 'narrows' of that tract (see Figure 1, page 36), where food slows down its passage and rubs against the intestinal linings most forcefully. (Occurrence of cancers at these points is significant when one notes how relatively long are the cancer-free portions of the intestine.) For cancer to occur in this fashion the irritation acts as a cancer promoter when the tissues are already in a pre-cancerous state. Irritation in the upper digestive tract (numbers 1–4) may be caused by hot food, certain condiments, and salt, and in the lower tract (numbers 5–10) by acids and toxins as well as hard compacted faecal matter resulting from constipation.

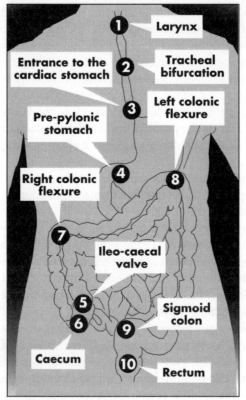

FIGURE 1. THE 'NARROWS' OF THE DIGESTIVE TRACT
Source: *Natural Food and Farming*, Atlanta, Texas.

THE SUNLIGHT CONNECTION

Exposure to sunlight will improve blood chemistry and circulation. Excessive exposure may damage the sub-surface skin cells of fair-skinned people, but whether such damage develops into a harmless self-healing skin lesion or a real skin cancer capable of malignancy will depend ultimately on the condition of the bloodstream and lymph fluid (the environment within).

THE SMOKING CONNECTION

Dr J A Scharffenberg, MD MPH, of California, in an article he wrote for *Life and Health* in 1979, provided statistics which showed that while mortality among smokers from cancer of the lung and throat was seven to ten times greater than that of non-smokers, it increased the risk of all other types of cancer as well by an average factor of two. At the same time, Dr Scharffenberg stated that the mortality from lung cancer in the USA had tripled since 1950 for both men and women and this was despite the fact that in that time the number of men who smoked had dropped from 60% to 40% and that, among women, only 29% smoked.

For lung cancer to increase in incidence three times while the number of people smoking decreased by one-third can only be explained again by pointing out the fact that it is the Western diet that has deteriorated since 1950, and although smoking is the killer it is claimed to be, the Western diet is a greater killer.

THE EXERCISE CONNECTION

If diet is the major factor in the causation of cancer, how does exercise convey protection against it? Exercise provides protection by improving the circulation and enhancing the immune system. The poorer the condition of the blood, the greater the importance of exercise.

Everyone knows that the heart is the pump that circulates the blood around the body, but less well-known is the fact that the return of the venous blood and of the lymph fluid in the tissues is largely dependent on the squeezing action on the veins that occurs with muscular movement, even the slight movements when asleep. When the blood is sticky due to high fat levels, the heart automatically pumps harder to increase the blood pressure, but the return circulation will be sluggish and, deprived of free-flowing supply of lymph, tissue cells — including brain cells — will be correspondingly handicapped. Thus even light exercise can be of great benefit, and the worse the condition, the more important the exercise becomes.

In the same situation (which applies especially to enthusiastic eaters), exercise of a more vigorous and sustained nature (aerobic exercise) provides even greater benefit because of the 'training effect' it produces after a while. When so 'conditioned', the body more efficiently utilises the excess fat from food and burns it up for energy. This is why athletes in condition display lower blood viscosity, lower blood pressure, lower cholesterol levels and more vigorous health than other people who consume the same sort of food as they do. It is not surprising that athletes, generally, experience only one-seventh the average incidence of cancer.

People who exercise regularly, even if they eat a Western diet, suffer less constipation, display lower levels of blood fats and cholesterol, lower blood pressure, and less hormonal abnormalities, thereby placing themselves in a safer position.

In 1985 a study by Dr R E Frisch compared the prevalence of breast cancer among women who had been athletes when at college with those who had not. He found that the non athletes had an 86% greater subsequent risk of breast cancer. A more recent study was undertaken in 1994, at the University of California under Dr Leslie Bernstein, involving 1090 women aged 36–40, half of whom had been newly diagnosed with breast cancer. The study found that moderate but regular exercise — four hours a week — reduced the risk of breast cancer by more than 50%.

WARNING

While physical fitness provides protection against cancer, heart disease, diabetes, arthritis and other problems by virtue of improving the circulation and enhancing the immune system, it cannot more than partially eliminate the toxaemia produced by improper diet and therefore the protection it provides is only partial.

Many athletes in intense training frequently are incapacitated by respiratory infections, due to the impairment of their immune systems caused by the intense stress of competition — mental as well as physical. Thus not a few such athletes have perished of cancer that otherwise may have remained static or perhaps not occurred in the first place.

THE STRESS CONNECTION

For centuries emotional stress has received a great deal of blame as a cause of cancer. As long ago as the second century AD, the famed Greek physician Galen attributed cancer to a melancholy disposition. The British surgeon Sir Heneage Ogilvie, writing in 1959, said:

> The instances when the first recognisable onset of cancer has followed almost immediately on some disaster, a bereavement, the break-up of a relationship, a financial crisis, or an accident, are so numerous that they suggest that some controlling force that has hitherto kept this outbreak of cell communism in check has been removed.

A lot has been written on this theme, but Dr Ogilvie's statement correctly sums it up. Stress at one time or another is an event a healthy body is equipped to deal with, and whereas a person may in indifferent health manage to live for years with pre-cancer or even 'controlled' cancer, trauma of a severe nature can upset their hormonal balance and diminish their immune system so severely that the hitherto controlled cancer breaks free.

Thus whether or not severe stress is successfully endured or whether it leads to grave illness depends upon the health status both mental and physical of the individual.

CONCLUSION

It all gets back to the conditions existing within the body — the condition of the environment within — the *milieu interieur*. You can call it simply 'body chemistry' or 'blood chemistry'. Whatever you call it the thing is to get it right, because then you will have homeostasis — freedom from disease.

Humans, in whatever part of the world they dwell, have a life potential determined mainly by the sort of food available to them, and to a lesser extent by external factors that further influence the composition of the environment within their bodies for better or worse.

Worry and stress can adversely affect the bloodstream, so can medical and other drugs (including oral contraceptives and oestrogen therapy), and so can smoking and alcohol. On the other hand, anti-coagulant drugs can protect against cancer by improving the blood circulation of chronically sick people.

So, in our own population, who gets cancer and who does not? For a start we know that currently 25% of all deaths are caused by cancer, but this does not mean that only one person in four gets it, the probability is that a large proportion of the other 75% of the population has pre-cancer or cancer but perishes of a heart attack or something else before the cancer becomes apparent. Autopsies show a lot of unsuspected cancer, so you cannot say the odds are very good.

In 1968 Dr G J Nossal stated that 22% of autopsies of non-cancer deaths reveal the presence of unknown malignancies. When in such autopsies the thyroid was investigated, over 50% contained malignant nodules. Other autopsy studies have shown that unsuspected cancer of the pancreas and thyroid is common, and prostate cancer is present in 50% of men over the age of 75 years. These observations were made 30 years ago, in the course of which time these cancers have become even more common.

Let us think positive. Who does NOT get cancer? Those who cancerproof their bodies.

CHAPTER 5

Some cancer theories

'There is no disease in existence which is, most assuredly,
easier of prevention than cancer; yet there is no malady which,
when once it has established its presence, is so difficult to subdue.'

— Robert Bell, MD FRFPS, Late Vice-president of the
International Society for Cancer Research,
Late Superintendent of Cancer Research at Battersea Hospital,
Member of the Cosmopolitan Society of Cancer Research

HOW AND WHY DO HEALTHY BODY CELLS CHANGE INTO CANCER CELLS?

Thus far the reader will have learned a lot about cancer and the various circumstances that lead to it. But how do these circumstances actually cause cancer? How do the many already known factors cause healthy body cells to change into cancer cells?

As was mentioned in the Introduction, in 1984 the ABC produced a TV program called *Understanding Cancer* in which various cancer specialists presented information on the subject of cancer and cancer research. The presentations were sincere and interesting but none of them went further than conjecture. As the experts themselves admitted, although a lot is known about the factors involved in cancer, it could not be satisfactorily explained how and why healthy cells sometimes change into cancer cells.

THE INJURY THEORY
Various theories have been put forward over the years, one of the earliest being that cancer was caused by injury such as a bruise or some form of irritation, because so frequently was it noticed that cancer arose in tissues so affected. However, this could never be explained, and of course in most cases of injury or irritation there is no cancer and normal healing ensues.

THE EMBRYO-CELL THEORY OF DR JOHN BEARD
In the late 1800s Dr Beard of Scotland observed that cancer cells resembled the undifferentiated cells of a growing embryo, sometimes being

indistinguishable from them. This led him to the conclusion that cancer originated from embryonic cells still contained in the body as undifferentiated left-overs from the embryonic state of the body's growth. Beard's theory never found acceptance — it being already known, at least by some doctors, that cancer cells were the offspring of normal cells which had, for reasons unknown, become abnormal.

THE VIRUS THEORY

Another theory — abandoned after the failure of the US Government's ten-year war on cancer (a war that cost more than ten billion dollars) — was the long-argued theory that cancer was caused by viruses.

This theory was based on the fact that, in the blood and tissues of cancer patients, viruses can be found that do not belong in healthy blood and tissues. However, this is also the case in many chronic conditions of disease, including AIDS, hepatitis, beriberi, and gangrene. The microorganisms present in the blood and tissues of these patients are accompaniments of the disease and not the cause of it, which explains why attempts to treat the problems with vaccines are not successful. It explains why news items of 'promising breakthroughs' always report promises and never successes.

THE INITIATION AND PROMOTION THEORY

One theory, which recognises the fact that a pre-cancerous condition exists before actual cancer appears, explains that carcinogenesis takes place in two stages: initiation and promotion. According to this theory various initiating factors alter tissues, so predisposing them to cancer, and that later on various 'promoters' take initiated tissue (but not normal tissue) a further stage to tumour formation.

This fundamentally correct theory is incomplete. It fails to explain the how and why of initiation and the how and why of promotion. It fails to explain the main event: why and how do healthy cells change into cancer cells?

THE DEFICIENCY DISEASE THEORY

A theory which is held to very strongly by many doctors researching the relationship between nutrition and cancer is that cancer is a disease caused by a deficiency of vitamins and minerals obtainable from green and yellow vegetables and fruit, primarily vitamins A, C, E and B17.

Whilst consistently it has been shown and is now generally accepted that such deficiencies contribute to the advent of cancer, it has never been shown that they alone can cause it and, moreover, no explanation has been tendered of the exact mechanism of how they could.

THE IMMUNE SYSTEM THEORY

Another theory still believed by many is that it is normal, even in healthy people, for cancer cells to be produced all the time only to be destroyed by the white cells of the immune system as a normal event, and that cancer only begins when the immune system breaks down.

While it is true that cancer patients display depleted immuno-competence, and that white cells tend to be antagonistic to cancer cells, the theory misses the point that it is not the break-down of the immune system that causes cancer: the break-down merely fails to arrest cancer already established.

THE MUTATION THEORY

Since the discovery of how various body characteristics and functions are controlled by genes in the DNA molecule of our cells, great enthusiasm has been applied to inventing theories of how various diseases are caused by the misbehaviour of one or more genes.

Ignorant of the fact that diseases such as arthritis, asthma, diabetes and multiple sclerosis have already been explained and successfully eliminated by natural means, medical research today still continues on the false assumption that these expressions of disease are aberrations brought about by misprogrammed genes and only correctable by 'scientific' medical procedures.

Cancer, according to this theory, is caused by a malfunctioning gene within a cell, and it is this malfunctioning gene that changes a previously normal cell into a cancer cell. It is assumed that only a single cell is so affected, and that from this one cell the cancer growth commences.

However, despite years of countless concentrated experiments, it has not been shown that human cancers occur in this way, although it has been claimed the gene responsible has been identified. It is called the 'onco-gene', but the way in which it is supposed to compromise a cell's mechanism to change it into a cancer cell cannot be satisfactorily explained, and therefore the theory remains only an unproven hypothesis. The hypothesis is a poor one from the start: if indeed a mutation was responsible for the changing of a normal cell into a cancer cell, then the subsequent progeny of that cell should, by the laws of heredity, all be the same, but they are not.

Dr Lucien Israel of France, in his book *Conquering Cancer*, states:

> In cancer, the reproduction of cells takes place in a highly abnormal fashion. It has long been known that, contrary to what occurs in healthy cells, when cancer cells divide, the number of chromosomes varies from one cell to another within the same tumour. The variations in time and space can be very great, the daughter cells do not necessarily contain an identical

number of chromosomes. There are many other visible anomalies, which are a nightmare for the specialists.

Even in pre-cancerous tissue, before the appearance of any true cancer cells at all, clearly detectable abnormalities, identifiable under an optical microscope, occur in numerous cells of the tissue, which — according to Drs Linus Pauling and Ewan Cameron — 'predict frank malignant change'. Thus it is obvious that numerous cells are involved, not just one, and that the only involvement genes have in the causation of cancer is that they are normal, performing at all times predictably in accordance with fixed biological laws, while ever the cells remain in a healthy state.

To say that the only involvement genes have in the causation of cancer is that they behave normally in a predictable manner is, of course, to invite heated rebuttal, because everyone knows that in pre-cancerous and cancerous cells the genes are *not* normal. There is no disagreement on that point, and there is no disagreement that a mutation of some sort rendered them abnormal. The point at issue is: what caused the mutation?

Medical researchers, having observed the abnormal genes within cancer cells, reacted as they once did when viruses were observed within cancer cells. The virus got the blame, then, for causing cancer. And now the abnormal gene is blamed. It is a short-sighted view. The crux of the matter is: what makes the genes abnormal in the first place?

The medical theory puts the blame for the mutation(s) on a hereditary factor; it goes so far as to say that cancer is unquestionably a hereditary disease.

Statistics show that the cancer risk among Greek migrants to Australia increases threefold within a few years of adopting Australian dietary habits. Have the Greeks' genes been changed by a change in countries? Of course not. It is their diet that has changed, and with it, the health of their cells.

The firmly held contention that a hereditary factor is involved in cancer is incorrect. Children have been born with cancer or with defects that predispose them to cancer, but such defects are congenital defects. These defects arise during the mother's pregnancy and are caused by poor nutrition or other lifestyle mistakes (such as drugs, smoking and alcohol). These are not inherited defects: they are injuries suffered before birth due to the appalling state of the mother's bloodstream.

CONCLUSION

Of the many carcinogenic substances known to be capable of producing cancer as demonstrated in laboratory experiments with animals, none have been shown to cause cancer in the concentrations to which humans are ever exposed. And although epidemiological evidence shows that without doubt many of these substances are frequently involved in human carcinogenesis, the mechanism of how and why remains essentially a mystery to the great majority of medical professionals.

Taking stock of the situation it becomes clear that without an understanding of the true cause of cancer, medical treatment of the disease cannot be successful. And that is a fact proven by the ever-increasing cancer death rate which has risen inexorably throughout the 20th century to account for one in four people and projected to account for one in three by the year 2000.

You might be thinking: if only the true cause of cancer was known, if only the true causes of asthma, arthritis, heart disease, diabetes and so on were known, what a blessing that would be! Not only could these 'diseases of civilisation' be successfully treated, they could easily be avoided in the first place.

Good news! The true causes of all these diseases are known and have been known for some years now. The diseases are reversible. They are preventable. You never need to fear them.

Diseases are not things that attack people — they are merely predictable reactions of the body to adverse conditions of blood chemistry caused primarily by eating the wrong kind of food.

The true cause of cancer is described in the chapter that follows.

CHAPTER 6

Explaining cancer

'Sit down before fact as a child. Be prepared to give up every pre-conceived notion. Follow humbly where Nature leads, or you will learn nothing.' — Thomas Huxley

MORE ABOUT CELLS

All forms of animal life require food and oxygen to provide their life energy. The food, in whatever form it is consumed, must first be digested of course, and broken down into basic chemical components that can be used by the cells of the body.

ENZYMES

Every process occurring within the body throughout life — from the digestion of food, the reassembly of the nutrients it contains, and the various uses to which the nutrients are put, the oxidation of blood sugar to provide cells' energy and so on — is dependent on the function of enzymes. Enzymes are complex chemical substances that act as catalysts to speed the various processes at the required, almost instantaneous, rate. Each separate chemical process of the thousands going on all the time requires a specific enzyme, and good nutrition is important to provide the body cells with the wherewithal to manufacture enzymes just as it is important to provide the body with its requirements to make blood sugar and protein. Thus there are thousands of different enzymes, many of which are concerned with the production of energy from the glucose in the blood.

THE EVOLUTION OF THE AEROBIC CELL

When life first appeared on Earth billions of years ago there was no free oxygen in the atmosphere. The first primitive life forms gained their energy by fermentation, which is a chemical process not requiring oxygen but at the same time is very inefficient.

When plant life evolved, plants gained energy from sunlight and sustenance from the earth and atmosphere, consuming carbon dioxide and liberating oxygen which had previously been locked up in other chemical compounds.

Until this time the first primitive animal cells were reliant on fermentation. With the availability of oxygen in the atmosphere, new cells began to evolve. These new cells, known as 'aerobic cells' (so called because they are dependent on oxygen), could gain energy from oxygen respiration, a much more efficient method. Whereas fermentation releases only a little energy (and leaves a residue of lactic acid, which is toxic), the aerobic cells using their new-found oxygen respiration could obtain 15 times the amount of energy from a given amount of food. Their oxygen respiration cycle still retained as part of it the primitive capacity of fermentation but was capable of intercepting the conversion of pyruvic acid to lactic acid and instead combining the pyruvic acid with oxygen to produce, as mentioned, 15 times the energy. An added advantage was that the only by-products were carbon dioxide and water, which are non toxic and useful to plants.

With the advent of the aerobic cell, evolution proceeded at an accelerated rate and eventually over aeons of time produced the forms of animal life, including humans, that inhabit the world today. Even fish living in water are dependent on oxygen, which they extract from the water passing through their gills. In polluted waters, fish and other marine life perish not only from poisoning but from oxygen deprivation.

Still existing today in various oxygen-deprived situations can be found primitive forms of life dependent on fermentation respiration, such as moulds and spores, which are anaerobic organisms and cannot tolerate normal levels of today's atmospheric oxygen. And still today there are aerobic organisms, such as various bacteria and other cell forms, which if deprived of oxygen are capable of reverting partly or even wholly to fermentation for survival, but in order to do so must change physically to a more primitive form. Some such organisms are capable of regaining their aerobic form if once again oxygen becomes available to them.

The evolution of plant and animal life-forms was a joint venture: plants constantly renewed the oxygen in the atmosphere, while animals used the oxygen combining it with carbon from their food to release it back to the plants as carbon dioxide. Thus all animal life-forms on Earth are entirely dependent on plant life, not only for oxygen but also for food.

Every cell in the human body in its normal condition is an aerobic cell reliant on the bloodstream and lymph fluid for food and oxygen to sustain it and to remove its waste products. Properly thus sustained and cleansed, all the cells remain in healthy condition and, in the absence of mental or physical trauma, homeostasis will prevail and disease will be impossible.

AEROBIC MICROORGANISMS

The human body is inhabited inside and out with numerous aerobic microorganisms. Some are bacteria that are essential to digestive processes, and some are germs that co-exist peacefully in our tissues. When homeostasis prevails, all is well, but when conditions within the body deteriorate many of these microorganisms can change in form to become pathological (that is, harmful), whereupon they can participate in worsening the state of health, and usually receive the blame for starting the sickness in the first place. Tuberculosis, hepatitis and the common cold are examples.

In understanding cancer it must be remembered that the aerobic cells making up all living creatures are fundamentally the same. Apart from their more complex DNA structure, the cells of the human body are no exception so that their individual reactions to any particular disturbance of their normal environment will be no different from that of the cells of more primitive life forms and even single-cell bacteria.

AEROBIC AND ANAEROBIC BACTERIA

An example of bacteria that can change in form should it become necessary, is the countless number of normal and harmless bacteria that inhabit our mouths. Under certain conditions these bacteria are capable of producing acid in the spaces between teeth, which corrodes the tooth enamel, causing decay. Why do the bacteria do this? They do it because certain kinds of food not ideally suited to the human diet (grain products are the worst) tend to block spaces between the teeth and deprive the bacteria there of oxygen. The bacteria, in an effort to survive, revert (de-differentiate) into an anaerobic form, in which form they can survive by fermenting the starch sugar. The by-product of their fermentation respiration is lactic acid, and it is the lactic acid which makes holes in the tooth enamel. Other primates in the wild don't have teeth problems because they have no option other than to eat the food provided by nature.

Another example of bacteria that change in form from aerobic to anaerobic respiration is the normally harmless bacteria which inhabit the human colon (bowel) and whose function is to break down food residues for excretion. If constipation occurs, the bacteria changes form.

Constipation (sometimes called intestinal stasis) is common in those who eat a Western diet. Cooked food is counterproductive to good digestion, and the sort of food that makes up a large part of the Western diet — meat and dairy products, and so on — is high in fat and cholesterol, low in fibre, and is difficult to digest. The incompletely digested residues remain often for several days in the colon, where they putrefy. The residues putrefy partly because they lack the fibre to give them bulk and because, being residues of an unnatural sort, the normal bacteria cannot properly function.

In the ensuing intestinal stasis the bacteria, deprived of oxygen, change in form to anaerobic bacteria, whereupon the fermentation they have become dependent on produces acids, gas and various toxins, some of which get into the bloodstream by way of the portal circulation.

Therefore it can be seen already how unsuitable food can cause problems at both ends of the digestive tract, but for the moment we shall continue discussing cell behaviour and return later to the rest of the dietary drama that happens in between the two ends.

DIFFERENTIATION AND DE-DIFFERENTIATION

The process of cell differentiation takes place in a developing embryo. At first, the cells are primitive in form; as they multiply, they gradually change into the different specialised cells required to construct the different organs of the baby's body.

At conception, when the egg and sperm unite to form one cell which then subdivides into two, then four, then eight, thus rapidly multiplying, the new cells — called 'embryonic cells' — all appear the same; they are primitive in form and are partially anaerobic and multiply rapidly without apparent constraint.

When the embryo attaches to the mother's circulatory system and begins to receive nourishment and oxygen from the mother's bloodstream, the embryonic cells become fully aerobic (dependent on oxygen). As the embryo grows, the cells multiply and begin to change in form: they become different from each other, and specialised, in order to construct the different organs of the baby's body, and growth slows down. The different cells become identifiable as bone cells, muscle cells, skin cells and so on, and when the process is complete the cells are said to be fully differentiated.

Normal embryo cells are initially primitive, undifferentiated, partly anaerobic, and multiply without constraint, whereas fully differentiated, specialised cells in normal tissues are fully aerobic and their subdivision and growth is strictly constrained.

De-differentiation

Under certain conditions it is possible for differentiated cells to become de-differentiated, which means that in the course of further cell division the new (daughter) cells undergo a change backwards towards a more primitive form — in other words, they tend to revert back in stages to the embryo form from which they descended. This is de-differentiation, and this is what cancer is all about.

HOW CANCER BEGINS

'Cancer, above all other diseases, has countless secondary causes. But, even for cancer, there is only one prime cause. Summarised in a few words, the prime cause of cancer is the replacement of the respiration of oxygen in normal body cells by a fermentation of sugar. All normal body cells meet their energy needs by respiration of oxygen, whereas cancer cells meet their energy needs in great part by fermentation' — Otto Warburg, double Nobel Prize Laureate, 1966

The information that follows in this section is based primarily on the research data and clinical experience of six of the most outstanding doctors of the 20th century: Drs Robert Bell, Otto Warburg, Dean Burk, William Koch, Max Gerson and Cornelius Moerman. Each of these doctors had over 50 years of clinical experience in the study of cancer and in the successful treatment of many patients given up as hopeless cases by ordinary standards. A great deal of data from other researchers with similar backgrounds is also included.

SIX OUTSTANDING DOCTORS

Dr Robert Bell

Dr Robert Bell, MD FRCS, was the leading cancer surgeon in England towards the end of the 19th century. His medical career spanned from 1870 to 1928. He was Vice-president of the International Society for Cancer Research, Superintendent of Cancer Research at Battersea Hospital, and Member of the Cosmopolitan Society of Cancer Research.

Dr Bell abandoned surgery in 1894 having realised the futility of excising a growth without attempting to correct the cause of it. He was thereafter constantly embroiled in controversy with the medical establishment. On one occasion he took court action to defend his reputation, as a result of which he was awarded damages of £10,000 (a lot of money in 1903). He was highly esteemed, despite his conflicts with the medical establishment, and was offered a knighthood by King Edward VII, an honour he declined.

Author of many books and medical research papers, his works included *Cancer, Its Cause and Treatment Without Operation, Health at its Best Versus Cancer, The Cancer Problem in a Nutshell, Cancer and Its Remedy, The Cancer Scourge and How to Destroy It* and *The Reminiscences of An Old Physician.*

As early as 1877 Dr Bell employed microphotography to observe the condition of patients' blood and the changes that occurred in tissue cells consequential to diseased blood. Upon his observations he was able to accurately describe the entire cancer process and explain it fully except for the factors involved in oxygen respiration, the discovery of which followed later and for which Dr Warburg was awarded his first Nobel Prize in 1931.

Dr Bell's description of the cancer process made a hundred years ago was the first accurate explanation of cancer and, although rejected at the time by the majority of doctors, was later proved correct by Dr Otto Warburg's discovery of oxygen transferring enzymes.

Dr Otto Warburg

Dr Otto Warburg (1883–1970), PhD MD, was Director of the Max Planck Institute of Cell Physiology in Germany. The holder of many international honours, Dr Warburg was considered by Dr Dean Burk, head of the Cytochemistry Department of the US National Cancer Institute at the time, to be the world's greatest biochemist.

In 1931 Warburg won the Nobel Prize in Medicine for his discovery of the oxygen transferring enzyme of cell respiration, and was voted a second Nobel Prize in 1944 for his discovery of the active groups of the hydrogen transferring enzymes. Conferred honorary degrees by the universities of Harvard, Oxford and Heidelberg, he was a member of the Royal Society of London, a Knight of the Order of Merit founded by Frederick the Great, and was awarded the Great Cross with Star and Shoulder Ribbon of the Bundesrepublik. Although Jewish, he was unmolested by the Nazis, and in the subsequent invasion of Germany by the Russians he was accorded protection and special consideration by the Russian High Command.

Warburg's research spanned more than 60 years, and he was the author of over 500 published research papers and five books. His description of the experiments in which he transformed normal cells into cancer cells was contained in his lecture at the meeting of Nobel Laureates on 30 June 1966 at Lindau, Germany. (This lecture is reproduced as Appendix A.)

Dr Dean Burk

Dr Dean Burk (1904–88), PhD, was a foundation member of the US National Cancer Institute and former head of its Cytochemistry Department. For his work in cancer research he received honours from France, Britain, Germany and Russia. Formerly Associate Professor of Biochemistry, Cornell University, he worked in cancer research at the Kaiser Wilhelm Institute in Germany and at the USSR Academy of Science, Moscow. Dr Burk was the recipient of the Domagk Prize for cancer research, a Knight Commander of the Medical Order of Bethlehem, and a Knight of the Mark Twain Society.

He was co-author of the books *Cancer, Approaches to Tumour Chemotherapy* and *Cell Chemistry* and author of over 250 published scientific papers.

Dr Warburg said Burk's outstanding and decisive discoveries in cancer research were: the metabolism of the regenerating liver (1941); that the malignancy of cancer was proportional to the fermentation rate of the cells

(1956); and that in vivo growing hepatomas produced in vivo by carcinogens were similarly more malignant the higher the fermentation rate (1964).

Dr William F Koch

Dr William F Koch, BA MA PhD MD, was Instructor in Histology and Embryology at the University of Michigan from 1910 to 1914, Professor of Physiology at the Detroit College of Medicine from 1914 to 1919, and Director of the Koch Cancer Clinic from 1919 to 1949. Like Max Gerson, Koch was considered unorthodox and a threat to the established medical system and, despite adoption of his methods by independent doctors in the USA and Canada, he was continually persecuted by the American Medical Association. The AMA was run at the time by a charlatan who called himself a doctor but whose medical credentials were false. This man's dictatorial control of American medicine finally ended when he was kicked out at the AMA Convention in Atlantic City on 6 June 1949.

Koch was author of numerous publications concerned primarily with the biochemistry of immunity and of cancer, his best known book being *The Survival Factor in Neoplastic and Viral Diseases*, published in 1961.

Dr Willard Dow, founder of the Dow Chemical Company, described Dr Koch as the greatest biochemist of the age and so far ahead of his contemporaries that they could not understand him.

Dr Max Gerson

Dr Max Gerson (1881–1959), MD, was Jewish but didn't enjoy Otto Warburg's standing. He was forced to flee Germany in 1933, and spent the last 20 or so years of his life working in the USA. Best known for his successful dietary treatment of migraine, lupus, tuberculosis, diabetes and cancer, Gerson was the author of more than 50 published research papers and four books, one of which, *A Cancer Therapy: Results of Fifty Cases*, should be essential reading for all medical students.

Whereas Warburg was supported and honoured for his full-time research, Gerson's great work was ignored by the medical establishment. He worked alone, devoting his efforts mainly to the treatment of his patients, most of whom had been given up as hopeless cases by other doctors.

Under Gerson's care, Dr Albert Schweitzer, double Nobel Laureate, completely eliminated his diabetes and, using Gerson's dietary method, Schweitzer's wife completely eliminated her tuberculosis. After Gerson's death Dr Schweitzer said of him: 'I see in him one of the most eminent geniuses in the history of medicine.'

Notwithstanding recognition by such medical greats as Dr Schweitzer and Dr Ferdinand Sauerbruch, Gerson's work received no recognition by the medical establishment, which considered him an unorthodox threat to the medical system.

The severest handicaps that prevented the general acceptance of Gerson's principles were: first, that having, with Sauerbruch's backing, been invited to address the Berlin Medical Society in 1933, he was forced to flee the Nazis only a few weeks before the scheduled meeting; secondly, the defeat in the US Senate in 1946 of a Bill to provide $100 million to coordinate research into Gerson's methods of treating cancer. Notwithstanding the testimony of many cured cancer patients, the Bill was narrowly defeated after intense lobbying from the AMA and vitriolic attacks on Gerson in the *Journal of the American Medical Association*, whose major source of revenue at the time was a cigarette company.

Nevertheless the continuation of Gerson's work by his daughter Charlotte, who is the leader of the Gerson Institute in California today, has more than anything else forced the medical establishment to think a little about nutrition.

Dr Cornelius Moerman

Dr Cornelius Moerman, MD, graduated in medicine in 1930 and then devoted his entire professional life to cancer research and treatment in Holland. His theory of cancer, which he called the Metabolism Theory, he developed independently, but because his reasoning was based on the new knowledge about the respiratory processes of cells and the enzymes necessary for their accomplishment, his conclusions inevitably coincided with those of Warburg, Burk and Koch (who were biochemists), and Gerson (who, like himself, was a physician).

The English translation of his book *A Solution to the Cancer Problem* was published in 1962 by The International Association of Cancer Victims and Friends, Los Angeles.

The novel way in which Dr Moerman developed his understanding of cancer is described in Chapter 8.

WHY AND HOW CANCER BEGINS

While it is claimed by some cancer specialists that cancer is not one disease but instead a hundred all under the one heading, others of equal standing say it is one disease but with many different manifestations. And yet none of these so-called experts can explain it.

So let us begin. All cancer cells, wherever they may be found, are the deformed offspring of once-normal cells and all have one vital common characteristic: they are all to a greater or lesser extent anaerobic, whereas all normal cells are 100% aerobic.

(There are no exceptions to this rule. In 1963 experiments in the USA appeared to have found an exception: the Morris Hepatoma, an extremely slow growing type of tumour. Further tests, by Drs Dean Burk and Mark Woods using more sensitive measuring equipment, proved that the Morris Hepatoma did indeed rely on fermentation to a slight degree, in keeping with its very slow growth rate, thus bearing out the fact that malignancy is proportional to the degree of anaerobiosis (fermentation) as indicated by the degree of lactic acid produced.)

Just as bacteria, which are single-cell organisms, can adapt to different degrees of oxygen deprivation by changing to partly anaerobic or fully anaerobic form, as necessary for their survival, so too can the cells of animal tissue. This fact provides the key to understanding cancer.

Normal aerobic cells will never change while their oxygen respiration remains intact but will tend to become anaerobic if oxygen respiration is curtailed. To do this they must revert to a more primitive state (that is, de-differentiate) with each cell division and, the more they are forced to do this, the less each generation of new cells is identifiable with the tissue cells of their origin, and the more each generation of cells becomes like primitive embryo cells capable of unrestrained growth. Thus cancer proceeds in degrees, with malignancy increasing proportionally with the degree of de-differentiation and the accompanying anaerobic process of fermentation — with its toxic lactic acid by-product — tightening the vicious circle.

It had long been known that cancer tissue displayed low oxygen concentrations when in 1966 Dr Warburg was able to measure these concentrations and thereby assess the degree of the tissue's malignancy. His measurements were as follows.

In healthy tissue, the ratio of anaerobic respiration to aerobic respiration was zero (because in healthy body tissue there is no anaerobic tendency at all); in healthy embryonic tissue, the ratio was 0.1 (that is, 9% anaerobic respiration); in benign tumours, the ratio was 0.45–1.45 (31%–59% anaerobic respiration); and in malignant tumours the ratio was 12 (92% anaerobic respiration).

In 1947 Dr F Windesch, also of Germany, demonstrated that by the intermittent withholding of oxygen, normal cells in vitro (in a test tube) could be changed into cancer cells. This demonstration was confirmed in 1953 by Drs H Goldblatt and G Cameron, and in 1966 Dr Warburg was able to measure the exact degree to which oxygen needed to be diminished in order to convert normal cells to cancer cells. He found that a 35% reduction of the cells' normal requirements of oxygen accomplished the change in the course of only two cell divisions in the space of 48 hours. (This is described in Appendix A.)

Typical human cancers do not occur rapidly like that, of course, even though their appearance and discovery may be sudden. The process is a creeping one — over many years and many cell divisions — and the oxygen deprivation, instead of being mechanically contrived in a bell-jar, occurs in other ways. Tissues may be poorly supplied with oxygen because of poorly circulating, sludged blood. Or even when adequate oxygen is available, mineral deficiencies may lead to diminution of the cells' respiratory enzymes; or the respiratory enzymes may be inhibited by toxins (carcinogens) from the bloodstream. One way or another, the final process is the same.

When comparing laboratory findings with what actually happens in the human body, an important difference to be borne in mind is that living cells once removed from their normal tissue automatically and blindly commence mitosis — the process of dividing which is necessary for de-differentiation to occur — whereas in the body the cell division of normal cells occurs only when needed and is strictly controlled.

In the body, cell division occurs most readily in the epithelial tissues (the tissues of the skin and of the membranes), and this is why 90% of lethal cancers originate in these tissues. Apart from the normal constant turnover of cells in epithelial tissues, it is these tissues which are most easily damaged either by injury, heat, chemicals or irritants, all of which lead to rapid cell division for healing (see Figure 1, 'The "narrows" of the digestive tract', page 36).

For healing to proceed, cells in the proximity of the damage must first of all de-differentiate in order to rapidly multiply, and this is why, when a pre-cancerous condition exists, tumours so often commence in such locations.

Thus the initiation and promotion hypothesis mentioned in Chapter 5, vague though it is, at least is on the right track. The pre-cancer is the initiation, and the injury or irritation is the promoter. The major and essential factor is the impairment of the cells' normal respiration in the first place, and the second requirement is the call for cell division, to which of course could even be added a third requirement: the failure of the immune system to arrest the cancer cells as they form. And so you can go on, but the fact remains that despite the conglomeration of factors that lead to pre-cancer and the variety of reasons for cell division, *there is, at the final accounting, only one primary and essential cause of cancer: the impairment of the tissue cells' oxygen respiration.*

It is likely that cancer often eventuates from pre-cancer anyway, without a promoter, because cells in epithelial tissue are renewed all the time, but in many cases the abnormal cells are arrested and destroyed by the immune system before they get out of control. That the immune system effectively controls cancer in its early stages there is no doubt, proven by the fact that cancer so often makes its appearance soon after the impact of severe emotional stress or physical trauma, which is well known to reduce immunocompetence. This is why people on immune-suppressing drugs following transplant operations so frequently come down with 'full-blown' cancer — an event which should not be surprising when it is contemplated that the conditions that made the transplant necessary would no doubt have already initiated the cancer well beforehand.

As biopsy and surgery call for cell division, and chemotherapy and radiation diminish the immune system, it would also be well to note that the conventional methods of treating cancer are effective methods of actually causing it when pre-cancer exists and causing metastasis from an existing primary tumour.

This is why surveys have shown that people who prefer to avoid medical treatment for cancer live longer and less traumatically than those who submit to treatment (more detail is provided in Appendix B).

FACTORS THAT AFFECT THE IMMUNE SYSTEM FAVOURABLY
- Natural diet
- Happiness and serenity
- High morale
- A positive attitude
- Adequate rest and sleep
- Fresh air and sunshine
- Physical exercise

FACTORS THAT AFFECT THE IMMUNE SYSTEM ADVERSELY
Most common
- Lack of factors listed above
- Toxaemia from dietary errors, constipation
- Dietary deficiencies, in particular vitamin C
- Worry
- Chemicals from different sources, including fluoride, chlorine and other chemicals in water supplies, and pesticide residues and other chemicals in food
- Medicine, including aspirin, tranquillisers and cough mixtures

More severe
- Alcohol
- Smoking
- Overweight
- Overwork, fatigue
- Mental trauma, including anger, pain, worry, frustration, grief and fear

- Physical trauma, including sexual excesses, excessive
  athletic training, prolonged discomfort, heat and cold
- Chemical trauma, including mercury in amalgam tooth fillings,
  poisons from infected teeth, poisons from insect bites and ticks,
  septicaemia, common medicines, prescription medicines,
  antibiotics and vaccinations

Very severe
- Severe malnutrition, such as from junk food, or from eating
  a diet that is high in sugar, salt, fat, and cholesterol, or from
  a severe vitamin C deficiency
- All drugs used habitually, whether taken intravenously,
  orally or inhaled, including marijuana and antibiotics
- Constant sexual promiscuity
- Receptive anal sex
- Bereavement, low self-esteem, feelings of guilt and hopelessness
- Mental trauma of voodoo or bone-pointing death sentence
  by shaman, witchdoctor, or modern physician

REGAINING HOMEOSTASIS

The importance of maintaining homeostasis in the body cannot be overemphasised, and as homeostasis does not exist in the body of someone with pre-cancer or cancer, every effort must be made to regain it.

All the vital organs are involved, of course, especially the liver and the kidneys and, because wear and tear on these two organs have more than anything else brought about the situation, they must be relieved of as much work as possible. Fasting is the most direct way to allow the body to regenerate; but, as deficiencies may be involved, the safest way is a diet that provides sustenance with the least amount of digestive effort and the least production of metabolic toxins. Dr Mackenzie Walser of the Johns Hopkins Clinic ascertained that, in the case of renal (kidney) failure, renal dialysis could be avoided — even if the renal capacity was only 2% — provided dietary protein was kept to a bare minimum on a diet of raw fruit and vegetables. The liver itself is capable of regeneration, so in this way it is possible for homeostasis to be restored and the body rebuilt.

As there may be no margin for error, new-found health should not be assumed to be a full recovery, and for some considerable time there may be little or no margin for error at all.

CANCER SUMMARISED

Cancer is a natural, predictable physiological reaction of normal healthy tissue cells to circumstances in their environment which inhibit their respiration of oxygen, forcing them to de-differentiate to a more primitive form reliant to a degree on fermentation to provide their energy needs. The degree of malignancy is determined by the degree to which the cells' oxygen respiration is curtailed and of necessity compensated for by further de-differentiation and increased fermentation, in the course of which each new generation of cells progressively comes to resemble the embryonic cells from which they are descended.

The circumstances in their environment referred to are collectively known as the cancer milieu, the explanation of which follows.

THE CANCER MILIEU

'A disease neoplasm, which cancer assuredly is, cannot possibly establish itself in healthy tissue.' — Robert Bell, *The Cancer Scourge and How to Destroy It*

Whereas Dr Otto Warburg summarised the prime cause of cancer to be 'the replacement of the respiration of oxygen on normal healthy body cells by the fermentation of sugar', I think it would be more correct to say that the replacement of cells' oxygen respiration by fermentation is more a description of what happens, while the actual cause of *why* this happens is the factor which in the first place deprives the cells of normal respiration and forces them to ferment if they are to survive. This factor is the cancer milieu: the polluted and inadequate milieu in which the cells are struggling to survive.

It may be asked how conditions within the body can affect healthy tissues to deprive them of oxygen in a manner anything like the laboratory methods of Warburg and others so to start the cancer process.

Before answering that question it should be understood that the restriction to a healthy cell's oxygen respiration does not cause *that* cell to de-differentiate — it influences that cell to divide into two daughter cells (mitosis) and it is these that are no longer fully differentiated. The two cells may be only slightly abnormal, and it may take many subsequent cell divisions in a worsening milieu before proceeding to cancer in the body. In the laboratory Warburg provided extreme conditions which produced cancer cells from healthy cells in only two subdivisions, but nevertheless it was the same process.

Although the cancer milieu exists throughout the entire body as a constitutional disorder, the condition of pre-cancer proceeds to cancer only when the affected cells are required to undergo cell division (mitosis), and for this reason primary cancer does not occur in tissues where there is no cell division.

Nerve cells do not undergo cell division, and cell division is infrequent in muscle cells. If circulatory conditions deteriorate enough, such tissues may ulcerate and proceed to gangrene and necrosis, but they do not produce primary cancer. Nerves and muscles can, however, support metastasised cancer (secondary cancer) which has found its way there from a primary elsewhere. Cell division, whether in normal tissue renewal or in the healing of injury or irritation, while an essential step in the formation of primary cancer, cannot be considered a cause of cancer, as cell division is a completely natural and normal occurrence.

Now to answer the question! How is the oxygen respiration of healthy body cells impaired by the cancer milieu?

The cells' oxygen respiration can be disturbed in several ways:

1. Diminished supply of oxygen due to sluggish circulation of sludged, sticky blood containing low concentrations of oxygen, circulation restricted by tight clothing.
2. By the absence of sufficient respiratory enzymes even when adequate oxygen is available.
3. By the inactivation or destruction of enzymes by carcinogens.
4. By a combination of these.

The extent to which each of these factors contributes to the problem must vary considerably, as will be evident in the discussion on the cancer milieu, but the opinions of Warburg, Koch, Gerson and Moerman tended to place the emphasis on enzyme impairment in the causation of primary cancer.

Dr Warburg considered the break-down of cell respiration to be due primarily to the absence of what he called 'active respiratory substances' inadequately supplied in the diet, and to a lesser extent, poor oxygen supply in the circulation. He thought that carcinogens were implicated by their effect of inhibiting the actions of the active respiratory substances. These substances included iron salts, riboflavin (vitamin B2), thiamine (vitamin B1), pantothenic acid, nicotinamide and cobalamin (vitamin B12).

Dr Koch said that clinical observations disclosed the persistence of toxaemia over a period as long as 20 years before the appearance of cancer. The eventual break-down in the cells' respiratory cycle occurred when various toxic amines de-activated the key respiratory components of the cell; he called these key respiratory components the 'functional carbonyl group' (FCG). Oxygen transport from the blood was reduced by poor circulation and gelation of tissue colloids, he said, but this alone without the deactivation of the FCG was not sufficient to cause cancer. Evidence of subsequent fermentation was the large elimination of lactic acid even when the lungs were well ventilated.

Dr Gerson divided the cancer process into two components: the general component and the local component. 'The general component,' he said, 'comprises mainly the deterioration of the essential organs of the digestive tract, chiefly the liver. There the damage is done by a permanent daily poisoning brought about by our modern civilisation.' The subsequent change in cells from normal to embryonic form, using fermentation, he ascribed to an inadequacy of oxidising enzymes and the presence in the cells of excessive sodium and a shortage of potassium. This is the local component.

Dr Moerman, like Dr Bell long previously, observed that cancer only appeared in tissues that were chronically sick, and said: 'In perfectly sound tissues, cancer has never yet to my knowledge come into being.' He said the factor that finally caused the break-down in cell respiration was injury to the oxygenating power of the cell due to the absence of nutritional substances such as vitamins A, C, B complex, and E, together with an absence of citric acid, iron, iodine, sulphur and others, in combination with an adverse sodium–potassium ratio.

It should be pointed out that all the opinions relate to the cause of cancer in its *primary form*, and that the metastasis of primary cancer involves different factors to do with the transport and settlement of already existing cancer cells. The following description of the cancer milieu should be considered with this in mind.

THE ROLE OF BLOOD SLUDGE AND BLOOD VISCOSITY

The bloodstream is called 'the river of life' for obvious reasons. Its function is to transport nourishment and oxygen to the tissue cells and to remove the cells' waste products for elimination. It is the job of the liver, with assistance from the other organs, to keep the blood pure and to furnish it with the various nutrients needed by the cells. It is the job of the heart to pump the blood around, and the job of the lungs to furnish oxygen to the blood as it passes through them. For all this to proceed properly the blood needs not only to be right in the chemical sense but also in the physical sense — it must flow freely.

Blood sludge and its associated viscosity (stickiness) is primarily due to excess dietary fat and protein, and in varying degrees is an almost universal problem because of the sort of food commonly consumed, and is made worse by alcohol, coffee, and so on, and again by both mental and physical stress. Medical drugs can also have an effect on sludging. (According to Dr Melvin H Knisely, some medical drugs cause sludging and others cause the blood to unstick.)

If the blood is sticky and sludged, the heart will need to work harder to maintain blood circulation — the effort, of course, will be reflected by the increase in blood pressure, but it is also common for many of the smaller blood vessels to become blocked for extended periods, so diminishing the supply of blood to the affected tissues. As the lymph (interstitial fluid), being part of the blood, is similarly handicapped, its function of cleansing the cells and removing their toxic wastes is curtailed. When cells are poisoned in varying degrees by their own wastes and poorly supplied with the oxygen and the nutrients they need, they get sick and the tissues degenerate.

Over one hundred years ago Dr Robert Bell's observations enabled him to state (from his book *The Cancer Scourge and How to Destroy It*):

> A disease neoplasm — which cancer assuredly is — cannot possibly establish itself in healthy tissue. It must, therefore, be assumed that before cancer can possibly occur in any locality, the health of the affected part has previously, to a greater or lesser extent, been seriously compromised.
>
> At this point I should like to draw attention to the fact that most valuable information may always be obtained by a careful examination of the blood; so much so indeed that the advent of disease of various kinds, and especially of cancer, may be recognised long before it has assumed an active stage of existence.
>
> It is therefore incumbent upon everyone who desires to guard against disease, to take every precaution to retain the vital fluid in its pristine healthy condition, and this objective can readily be attained by conforming to those hygienic laws, which is the duty of everyone, who is the possessor of a well-balanced mind, to make himself thoroughly acquainted with, and obey to the letter.

Over the past 30 years Dr Leopold Dintenfas of Sydney has made an exhaustive study of blood viscosity and its role in many diseases. Quoting from Dr Dintenfas's several books:

> The high viscosity syndrome can contain one, two, or more elements [the elements that influence the viscosity of blood are plasma viscosity, aggregation of red cells, haemoconcentration, aggregation of platelets, and concentration of white cells]. Capillary occlusion, stasis hypoxia, acidosis, necrosis, and infarction are inevitable, although not necessarily irreversible steps in this process.
>
> It would be worthwhile to note that osteo and rheumatoid arthritis are associated with an elevation of plasma viscosity and an elevation of the degree of aggregation of red cells. High blood viscosity always leads to a slowdown of circulation and to reduced oxygenation of tissues.
>
> Wardle in 1976 suggested that it is the increased blood viscosity in the small digital arteries which is responsible for the common symptom of malignancy. Red cell aggregation, platelet aggregation, and hypercoagulability can contribute to this syndrome. Crenated red cells, raised fibrinogen, increased platelet stickiness are all a common feature of malignancy.

That poorly circulating sticky blood is a major factor in the onset and progression of cancer there can be no doubt at all, and is confirmed by the fact that the erythrocyte sedimentation rate (ESR) is almost invariably high in all cancer patients.

Further confirmation that high viscosity blood may lead not only to primary cancer but also to metastasis of primary cancer, was provided by Dr Summer Wood of Boston in 1958. He demonstrated that for metastasis to occur, stray cells from a primary tumour must first avoid destruction by the immune system and then lodge in a location where the circulation is blocked by a thrombosis (fibrin clot).

The role of exercise in relation to blood viscosity

Further confirmation that poorly circulating sticky blood is a major factor in the onset and progression of cancer comes from the knowledge that, all other things being equal, fit athletes experience only one-seventh the incidence of cancer, and this is attributable to the fact that their blood viscosity remains low due to the training effect which readily metabolises blood fat for fuel, and also to the effect of exercise stimulating the circulation.

To again quote Dr Dintenfas:

Studies of athletes, normal individuals, and patients with cardiac and renal diseases show a progression from a low blood viscosity with a high flow velocity among athletes, to an elevated viscosity and low flow velocity among patients. Furthermore, my colleagues and I have found time and again an elevation of blood viscosity among apparently healthy individuals who later developed symptoms of heart disease and cancer.

Anti-coagulants

About the same time as the observations of Dr Summer Wood, Dr L Michaels of Canada reasoned that if no clots were allowed to form, then metastasis could not occur, and that people with only primary tumours would in that case be in a much safer situation. This proved to be the case. He studied the medical histories of a large number of heart and stroke patients kept on permanent anti-coagulant drug treatment to protect their blood circulation, to ascertain the incidence of cancer deaths among them, and found the incidence to be only one-eighth of the expected number. The study covered the equivalent of 1569 patient-years and there was not a single case of death by cancer metastasis in the group.

A similar study by Dr Bjorn Stinkvist, University Hospital, Upsala, Sweden, on women maintained on digitalis for cardiac problems, showed that spreading breast cancer was only one-tenth the rate experienced by women not on digitalis, and even when it occurred the cancer was less aggressive.

It is easy to see why fat is a major factor in most cancers and why herbal anti-coagulants (such as garlic, aloe vera, and so on) assist people to avoid cancer and heart attacks. Dr Gerson in his book *A Cancer Therapy* said that: 'the rare incidence of malignant tumours in countries where garlic is used in greater amounts (Southern Italy, Greece, Montenegro, Yugoslavia) cannot be explained'. Today, however, we can easily explain the role of garlic: it counteracts the excess fat in the blood, thinning it out so that the blood flows easier. This is why garlic is so effective in relieving circulatory problems and lowering blood pressure of people consuming a high fat diet.

Further supportive information to do with the importance of maintaining free circulation is provided by Dr Dintenfas in his book *Rheology of Blood in Diagnostic and Preventative Medicine*:

> Olwyn (1971) in his editorial, reviewed the effect of anticoagulants on tumour metastasis and noted that a number of investigators found a significant protection from metastasis by the application of [anticoagulant therapy]. In an informal survey of 200 patients with a history of myocardial infarction or cerebral arterial insufficiency receiving [anticoagulant treatment] for periods of two to twenty-two years, Griffith (1971) found no instance of malignant tumour. Michaels (1971) who reviewed 540 patients on oral anticoagulant therapy for thrombo-embolic disorders, found presence of metastasis reduced eight fold against statistical expectation.

Final proof

The final proof of the pudding regarding the connection between blood flow and cancer could well be the fact that primary cancer so very rarely occurs in the liver, despite its being the body's first line of defence against carcinogens and the most exposed to them. As well, the liver is capable of rapid reproduction of new cells just like the epithelial cells. Despite these two potentials for cancer, primary tumours of the liver account for only about 1 in 200 of the total, and the reason for this apparent anomaly must surely be that the liver has the most assured and profuse blood supply in the body.

However, the animal experiments have shown that, even with adequate circulation, cells' aerobic respiration can be readily impaired also by the absence or impedance of the necessary respiratory enzymes, and the extent to which each factor contributes to the cancer milieu no doubt varies considerably. No matter, the object of the exercise is to eliminate both factors: the high blood viscosity and the impaired blood chemistry associated with it, so to restore homeostasis in the body.

THE ROLE OF TOXAEMIA

Toxaemia is a poisoned condition of the blood and can exist in varying degrees. Burdened with fat particles that enter the blood in large quantities from fatty meals, as well as with toxic substances, the blood condition is called 'lipotoxaemia' ('lipo' means fat). Sticky blood is bad enough, but with the addition of toxic by-products from the digestion of various unsuitable food-stuffs common to the Western diet, the blood becomes toxic as well as sticky.

Many people think of toxaemia as being caused by contaminants contained in food — preservatives, colouring agents, artificial flavourings and so on — and by various chemicals inhaled, digested, or absorbed through the skin, all of which are derived from outside the body (that is, they are exogenous substances). But whereas these substances may cause minor health problems, there is a source of toxins far worse. The toxaemia that is by far the most potent in the genesis of cancer comes by way of toxins produced from within the body (endogenous toxins).

Some toxins are produced in a healthy body as a normal event all the time, as by-products of digestion and as the waste products of all the cells, but the blood is quickly purified by the liver and kidneys, with the toxins sent to the bladder to be expelled. Toxaemia can only occur if the level of toxins exceeds the capability of the liver and the kidneys to accomplish their job. On a natural diet the amount of toxins produced is little, and the liver has no problem in maintaining homeostasis.

On the Western diet high in protein, cholesterol and fat, mostly cooked and salted, the level of body-made toxins is so high that the vital organs are constantly overworked to maintain homeostasis. Good health lasts as long as homeostasis is maintained but as people get older and their vital organs begin to weaken, homeostasis may from time to time (or perhaps all the time) be lost, following which toxaemia increases and the diseases of civilisation make their appearance.

The most dangerous toxins produced in the body, and the ones which are most carcinogenic when taken into the main bloodstream, are those produced in the colon (large bowel). On a natural diet there would be none of these, but on the Western diet, the unexpelled, incompletely digested residues of cooked protein and fat containing no fibre to assist their passage, ferment and produce toxic acids and chemicals which are absorbed by way of the portal circulation into the main bloodstream. (Constipation will be discussed in Chapter 7.)

Infected teeth poison the bloodstream

Another source of endogenic carcinogens are infected teeth, and these toxins can be a major contributor to the cancer milieu. Dr Mulhim Hassan of

Lebanon has devoted most of his long medical career to the study and treatment of cancer. In his book *Prevention and Cure of Cancer* he emphasises that poisoning of the bloodstream by toxins from diseased teeth is a common and potent factor in a great many cases of cancer. His book is illustrated with many photographs showing the healing of various cancers subsequent to the removal of the oral focuses of infection.

Another famous cancer specialist, Dr Joseph Issels of Germany, now in Florida, has for 50 years asserted the same argument, insisting that the removal of infected teeth be the very first thing to be attended to in cases of cancer. Another German doctor, Dr Max Garten agreed: 'This is one phase in cancer treatment that requires adamant and uncompromising attention.'

THE ROLE OF DEFICIENCIES

Everybody knows how important it is to get enough vitamins and minerals in their diet. Without the full range of these essential components of food, all the rest is wasted, the body cannot function. Nor can it function without enzymes, of which the body makes thousands, because it is enzyme action of one kind or another that is involved in every process that takes place in the body. Without enzymes there would be no life on Earth of any kind. Without the right nutrients in the diet the body may not be able to make all the enzymes it needs. To maintain aerobic respiration requires the proper respiratory enzymes, and a shortage of these of course will contribute to the cancer milieu, whether the shortage be caused by a dietary deficiency or by the destructive action of carcinogenic toxins.

LIVER DEGENERATION

Whereas it has commonly been shown in the laboratory that grossly applied methods can quickly bring about cancer, either by the straight-out withholding of oxygen from cells or by the straight-out application of poisonous chemicals, it may be argued that humans are never subjected to such conditions and that the animal experiments are of no value. However, when the time factor is taken into account, the experimental findings are immensely instructive in so far as they do indicate what happens in real life, slowly and over a long period, when various factors combine to achieve the same result.

What animal experiments do show clearly is the vital fact that whatever the methods used to administer carcinogenic chemicals to the animals, cancer never makes its appearance while the liver is reasonably functional. Only when the liver is sufficiently damaged by the chemicals is any kind of cancer possible. As Dr Gerson pointed out:

The experimental causation of cancer, first accomplished by Yamagiva and Itchikawa, through rubbing tar substance on the ears of rabbits for about nine months, is of importance in so far as they found that before the cancer started to appear, the liver was damaged and showed pathological changes, together with the kidneys, spleen and the lymphatic apparatus. The long period was required to poison the liver, before the damaged cells could form the 'mutation' into cancer.

Further proof that the cancer resulted from the poisoning of the bloodstream and not from the *local* effect of the tar on the ears of the mice was provided when cancer made its appearance at the site of a cut made elsewhere on a mouse's body and not at the expected point where the tar had been applied. The mouse's tissues were pre-cancerous, and the cancer itself followed the ensuing subdivision of cells required for attempted healing of the injury. Further proof, again, was provided by an experiment of Dr Gerson's in which the circulatory systems of a cancerous rat and a healthy rat were interconnected, whereupon the cancer in the sick rat diminished and then disappeared. (Such mixing of bloodstreams is possible only when blood is perfectly matched, as occurs in identical twins and as occurred in the entire strain of these laboratory rats.)

Cancer used to be called 'the disease of the aged', but as the nutritional quality of the modern diet continues to decline, the eligibility for cancer extends now to younger age groups. With the advent of supermarket provisioning and the increased dependency on packaged, canned and processed food — and the advent of take away pizzas, fried chicken, and hamburgers loaded with fat and salt — people's digestive organs, notably the pancreas, kidneys and liver, start packing up sooner than they used to, so that sickness care (the government calls it 'health care') has become the nation's number-one problem.

CHAPTER 7

More on diet and other factors

'The three major killers in modern society, Coronary Heart Disease, Cancer and Strokes, can all be linked to what people eat and drink.'
— Dr B Hetzel, Chief of the CSIRO Division of Human Nutrition, and Foundation Professor of Social and Preventative Medicine, Monash University

Generally speaking, the incidence of cancer around the world is proportional to the degree of sophistication and technical development attained by different population groups, particularly in regard to food selection and food preparation. However there are probably thousands of other man-made factors that in one way or another tend to worsen people's body chemistry and help to predispose them to cancer and these should all be taken into account, but in light of all the evidence, their contribution must be considered minor compared to the auto-intoxication that people create within their own bodies.

Whether or not the explanation of cancer as set out in the preceding chapters is clearly understood by the reader, there is one fact that can no longer be disputed: *the prime, essential factor in all common human cancers is faulty diet*. Sufficient proof of this was provided in the findings of Dr Summer Wood and Dr Michaels (mentioned in the preceding chapter), that cancer, both primary and secondary, was prevented in very cancer-prone people simply by thinning their blood with anti-coagulant drugs. The same thinning of the blood is even more simply achieved by the adoption of a completely natural diet, which at the same time clears the system of toxaemia as well, thereby *doubling* the protection.

Dr Jeremiah Stamler's report on a study of 100,000 Seventh Day Adventists provides additional insight. The study emphasised dietary habits and was conducted about 20 years ago by the Loma Linda University, California. It showed that their cancer rate (all kinds) was only half that of the national average. A similar study of 800 Adventists in Sydney, about the same time, showed the incidence of common cancers such as lung and stomach cancers was only one-third that of the rest of the community, and the incidence of abnormal blood pressure and high cholesterol was only one-tenth. But more revealing again were the comparisons made within the ranks of the Adventists themselves, who comprised non-vegetarians as well as total vegetarians. The death rate of the total vegetarians from all the diseases was less than half the death rate of the non-vegetarians.

Further proof that the essential factor in all common human cancers is faulty diet is provided, of course, by the natural 'spontaneous remissions' of established cancer achieved by dietary means after the failure of conventional medical treatment. (Spontaneous remission is described and explained in Chapter 9.)

THE ROLE OF FAT

Excess dietary fat plays the major role in all the diseases of civilisation and particularly in cancer.

The human system is not equipped to cope with cooked or processed fat. Animal and vegetable fat is mainly consumed in cooked form, and it is in this form that it is most harmful: difficult to digest, destructive to the vital organs and disruptive to the body's chemical balance. Incompletely broken down by the struggling digestive organs, a great deal of fat bypasses the liver and enters the lymph system and then into the main bloodstream and, by its physical presence in the blood, it increases the blood viscosity (stickiness). The red blood cells stick together, so do the blood platelets, and the white

---

DIETARY FATS

The fat requirements of the human system are best supplied by free fatty acids contained in natural fruits and vegetables whereby a total fat intake of about 4% of total calories is provided, as against 40% (of the wrong kind) in the Western diet. When reducing dietary fat, little benefit is gained until fat is reduced below 20%; best results are gained at less than 10%. Only the strictest of diets can achieve this figure.

Fats of the right kind are the mono-unsaturated fats contained in avocadoes and olive oil (best in the raw state), and the super-unsaturated (omega 3) fats contained in fish. These fats, when incorporated in the Western diet, are favourable to blood circulation (as with garlic) and are therefore protective.

Fats of the wrong kind include polyunsaturated oils and margarine, surveys having shown that the increased consumption of polyunsaturated fats increases the risk of cancer, a fact that has been confirmed in animal experiments.

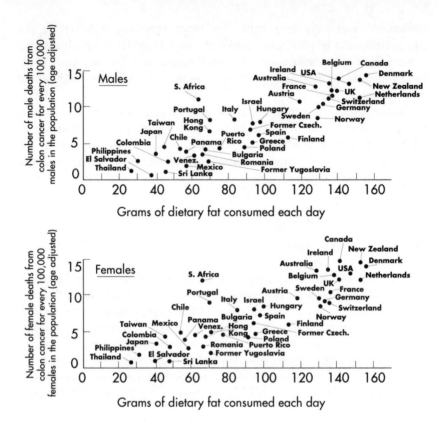

FIGURE 2. DEATHS FROM COLON CANCER IN RELATION
TO DAILY CONSUMPTION OF ANIMAL AND VEGETABLE FATS
Source: Kenneth K Carroll, 'Experimental evidence of dietary factors
and hormone-dependent cancers', *Cancer Research*, vol. 35, p. 3379.

cells of the immune system are similarly handicapped, the heart's workload
is increased, blood pressure increases while at the same time circulation in
some areas is diminished or shut right off. Mental processes slow down.

THE INFLUENCE OF FAT UPON HORMONE PRODUCTION

Another dangerous effect of a high fat diet is that it increases the production
of the female growth hormone oestrogen, elevated levels of which are
associated with the appearance of lumps and cysts in the breast — which
frequently precede breast cancer — and, once cancer has appeared, high
levels of oestrogen accelerate its growth. The incidence of breast cancer
brought about this way in countries with high fat consumption is very
great; for instance, the Dutch and the Danes have seven times the

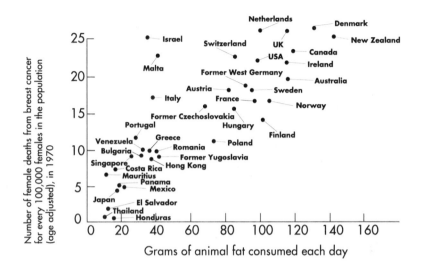

FIGURE 3. DEATHS OF FEMALES FROM BREAST CANCER
IN RELATION TO DAILY CONSUMPTION OF ANIMAL FATS
Source: Kenneth K Carroll, 'Experimental evidence of dietary factors and hormone-
dependent cancers', *Cancer Research*, vol. 35, p. 3379. (Similar graphs have
been separately prepared from statistics for skin cancer and prostate cancer
as related to fat consumption. They show the same relationship.)

rate as the Japanese, whose low fat diet protects them also from bowel
cancer and lung cancer.

It is because of the high fat levels in the modern diet that the increased
oestrogen brings about the premature sexual development in young girls
when compared with past eras, and the general demand for larger
sized bras. And talking about bras, they are suspected of contributing
to breast cancer in some cases where bras have been tight enough to restrict
blood circulation.

In research findings by Professor Hermann Aldercreutz of Helsinki
University Hospital, a high fat diet caused increased levels of male
growth hormones as well as female growth hormones, and these
increased levels were directly related to prostate cancer in males as well
as to breast and bowel cancer. Offsetting to a certain degree these adverse
effects was a greater intake of dietary fibre.

A report from the Meyer L Pentis Comprehensive Cancer Centre of
Michigan, published in 1994, showed that dietary fat stood out as the major
factor in prostate cancer.

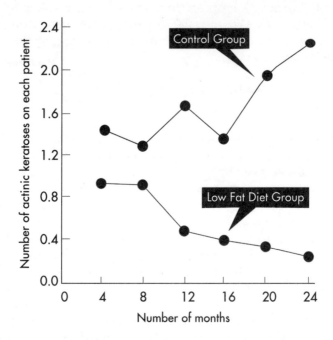

FIGURE 4. DIET AND SKIN CANCER: THE INCIDENCE OF ACTINIC KERATOSIS
(PRECURSOR OF SQUAMOUS CELL CARCINOMA) MEASURED AT FOUR-
MONTH INTERVALS IN A CONTROL GROUP AND A LOW FAT DIET GROUP
Source: H S Black et al., *New England Journal of Medicine*, vol. 330,
no. 18, May 1994, pages 1272–5, cited in *Vantage Point*, vol. 4, no. 8, 1994.

It would be incorrect to assume an excess of hormones is a cause of cancer because, unless a pre-cancerous condition existed already, their influence would be merely to encourage growth of healthy tissue. However, in the event of pre-cancer or cancer, the hormones would act as cancer promoters. One way or another, abnormal levels of hormones or anything else are undesirable.

The pill and oestrogen therapy

Whereas the cancer-promoting influence of excessive levels of oestrogen is mainly attributable to dietary fat, there is a great deal of evidence that additional oestrogen from oral contraceptives and hormone replacement therapy (HRT) add further to the risk. This should not be surprising.

Research at the Netherlands Cancer Institute under the direction of Dr Matti Rookus found: 'We conclude that four or more years of pill use, especially if before age 20, is associated with an increased risk of breast cancer at an early age. Our findings strongly suggest long term oral contraceptive use is related to the risk of breast cancer.' (Further information will be found in Appendix C.)

THE INFLUENCE OF FAT UPON SKIN CANCER

None of this information is new: it has been recorded for at least 30 or 40 years.

A report published in 1994 described the results of a 24-month trial on 76 patients with a history of non-melanoma skin cancer. Researchers at the Baylor College of Medicine, Houston, divided the patients into two groups: one group was put on what was called a 'low fat diet' (20% of kilojoules/calories from fat) and the other, a control group, ate a typical American diet (40% fat). The incidence of crusty lesions called 'actinic keratosis', which are precursors of carcinomas, was recorded. The 20% fat group at the end of the trial recorded an incidence of lesions of 0.25 per patient compared with 2.3 in the high fat group — only one-ninth the number! (See Figure 4.)

It should be noted that, as will be shown in Chapter 10, a 20% fat diet is still way too much fat for optimum health, and therefore with a more drastic reduction of fat the incidence of lesions would be reduced probably to zero.

THE INFLUENCE OF FAT UPON BRAIN FUNCTION

Environmentalists are seeking to outlaw leaded petrol which they claim to be a factor in the diminished IQ of many children due to lead particles released from vehicles into the atmosphere. They should pay greater attention to the perils of the Western diet!

Nathan Pritikin described years ago how children whose diet was changed from the typical Western diet to a diet low in fat could, after a few days, perform simple mental arithmetic 20% faster and with fewer mistakes once their blood was clear of fat. This explains why children of Asian migrants out-perform other children: they inhale the same amount of lead, but as yet do not take in the same amount of fat.

All age groups are fat-handicapped. To again quote Dr Leopold Dintenfas:

A hypothesis by Walsh is that presenile dementia is a result of arterial insufficiency of the brain consequent to thrombotic processes in the arteries supplying the brain. This hypothesis is reinforced by the findings of Alvarez that senile and presenile dementia is often preceded by 'little' strokes. Walsh showed that presenile and senile dementia can be prevented by anticoagulant therapy, thus substantiating the fact that mental disorders might be a direct result of occlusive circulatory disorders.

A typical case demonstrating this to be true is one described in an early newsletter of the Pritikin Longevity Centre:

> Senility — 83 year old male with increasing senility in the last year so that he was unable to communicate, walk by himself, and maintain toilet control. By the end of the four week session he had completely regained his mental faculties and carry on a spirited conversation. His ability to walk by himself returned and he experienced a substantial return of other lost functions.

Thus it is clear that diminished mental acuity due to the Western diet is a problem not only to be measured in children, and it would be interesting to observe the effect on our country's fortunes if the dining rooms in the nation's capital were converted to fruit-juice bars.

CONSTIPATION (INTESTINAL STASIS)

Not only does the Western diet directly cause blood pollution and high blood viscosity, it is guaranteed also to cause constipation, from which further blood pollution ensues. In most respectable homes can be found, along with all the other patent medicines, some form or other of bowel-opening preparation, and perhaps one or two magazines in the bathroom.

For over a hundred years it has been observed by doctors that the most common factor associated with all forms of cancer is the condition of constipation. The British surgeon Sir William Arbuthnot Lane (1856–1943) repeatedly emphasised that he had never known a single case of cancer which had not been preceded by prolonged intestinal stasis.*

Professor Aviles, of the Biochemistry of Cancer Department,Guadalajara, Mexico, found that out of 7715 cancer patients examined over a 15-year period, 99% had suffered from constipation and that the degree of malignancy was parallel to the degree of constipation.

---

* William Arbuthnot Lane, BART CB, was Consulting Surgeon to Guy's Hospital, Consulting Surgeon to the Hospital for Sick Children in London, President of the New Health Society, and author of *The Prevention of the Diseases Peculiar to Civilisation* (1929). In his surgical practice, Sir William noted that so common were diseased colons, he was forced to conclude the colon to be the seat of most chronic diseases, and for some time he specialised in the removal of diseased colons. This procedure confirmed his ideas because most of his patients' chronic disorders cleared up very quickly after losing their colons, and their overall health improved. Eventually he realised the colon was not, itself, a troublesome organ, that it became diseased only because of the kind of food people ate, and that the resulting disorders were the result of what he called 'auto-intoxication'. It was at this time in his career he became converted to the concept of natural health and thereafter concentrated his efforts on educating patients rather than cutting pieces out of them.

A LESSON FROM RURAL AFRICA

Dr Denis Burkitt and Dr Hugh Trowell of England both spent 25 years as doctors in areas of rural Africa. These doctors observed over that time that constipation in these areas was virtually non-existent, and so too was cancer. Dr Burkitt noted that the rural Africans passed about one pound of faecal matter each day, about four times the amount of English people, and that the Africans' faeces were soft, bulky and almost odourless.

Investigation showed another significant thing. The transit time from eating to elimination was for the African about 24 hours, whereas with the English it was three days or more. This meant that, even with a daily bowel movement, the wastes of food eaten by the English remained within them three times as long.

The obvious cause of these differences was the sort of food eaten. The average African villager ate mainly cornmeal, beans, bananas and potatoes. This diet was low in fat and animal protein, devoid of refined carbohydrate, and contained about three times the amount of vegetable fibre of the English diet.

The researchers analysed countless medical records and this is what became evident:

1. Cardiovascular disease, the leading cause of death in Western countries, was virtually unknown in rural Africa.
2. The cancers of Western populations were also virtually unknown.
3. Diabetes, hypertension, appendicitis, haemorrhoids, diverticulitis, varicose veins, phlebitis, obesity and hernias were also virtually unknown.

As Dr Tipper said, in reference to West African tribesmen: 'There is no such thing as constipation and there is no cancer. At the first dawn of civilisation amongst them, the disease makes its appearance; where civilisation is advanced, it is rife.'

THE WESTERN DIET IS CONDUCIVE TO CONSTIPATION, AND THEREFORE TO CANCER

The Western diet not only causes lipotoxaemia and high blood viscosity by virtue of excess fat, cholesterol, protein and so on entering the system directly from the digestion, but in addition causes auto-intoxication when unexpelled wastes putrefy in the colon (large bowel).

THE ROLE OF BACTERIA IN DIGESTION

The digestive process involves bile from the liver and the action of bacteria normal to the colon. These bacteria comprise 20–30% of the bulk of the faeces.

There are different types of colon bacteria. Healthy people have a type which require oxygen to live, called 'aerobic bacteria'. With a low fat, high fibre diet, normal aerobic bacteria operate free of toxins, the high fibre faeces contain a much higher proportion of intact bile, and the faecal matter stays in the colon less than 18 hours, as studies by Dr M G Hall of the Bacterial Metabolism Research Laboratory, London, have shown.

On the other hand, with the putrefying remains of a high fat, high protein, low fibre diet, the bacteria change to a form of anaerobic bacteria, which take over the colon, and these react with acids in the bile to form poisons, which include apcholic acid and deoxycholic acid which are carcinogenic. Not only is the colon therefore constantly exposed to these carcinogens in an oxygenless situation, but at the same time the toxins are taken up by the bowel veins and so enter the already polluted bloodstream to exert their carcinogenic effect throughout the entire body.

The Western diet is further conducive to cancer in that it lacks not only the necessary fibre but lacks also the anti-carcinogenic substances contained in the missing raw fruit and vegetables.

SQUATTING VERSUS SITTING

Squatting is the easiest, most natural and healthiest position for defecation. (It is also the most natural position for giving birth.)

One reason for the chronic constipation among Western populations is the use of the pedestal toilet. (A brief history of the pedestal toilet, by William Welles, DC, is provided as Appendix E.)

Population groups who traditionally use floor-level toilets, and those who use the great outdoors, do not suffer constipation like Westerners do. For this reason in health magazines you can see advertised plastic contraptions designed to fit over the conventional pedestal bowl so that you can squat, albeit some distance above the floor.

The plumbing of the human anatomy is arranged to work in the squatting position. When a person squats to defecate, the recto-anal angle at the end of the anal canal straightens out to permit easy evacuation; whereas, if a person sits, the sharper recto-anal angle forms a constriction and so pressure is required to force the contents of the bowel though it.

Other problems associated with constipation, such as haemorrhoids, prostate inflammation, cystitis, backaches and incontinence, are also avoided or relieved by adoption of the squatting position.

The importance of the ileocaecal valve and the appendix

Apart from the seated position making evacuation more difficult, the constant exertion of muscular pressure within the colon is damaging to the ileocaecal valve, which is located between the intestine and the colon and serves to prevent the colon's harmful substances and bacteria returning to the intestine (which is sterile). (Refer to Figure 1, 'The "narrows" of the digestive tract', on page 36).

Further protection to the intestine is provided by the appendix. As described by Dr Norman Walker in his book, *Colon Health*, the appendix secretes a powerful germicidal fluid. This germicide acts as a barrier protecting the intestine from the entry of colon bacteria, and likewise protecting the colon from any harmful substance entering it from the intestine. (So constant sometimes is the demand upon the appendix that it may lose function and become inflamed by poisons and harmful bacteria from the colon, causing appendicitis.) Eventual weakening of the ileocaecal valve further diminishes this protection and permits toxins from the colon to enter the intestine and add to further deterioration of the bloodstream.

A LESSON FROM THE NAVAJO

An illustration of the importance of squatting is provided by Dr De Lamar Gibbons's study of North American Indians in San Juan County. In 32 years of practice, Dr Gibbons noted that despite the Navajo's appalling diet (containing large amounts of fat and junk food, and no vegetables), cancer was almost non-existent, although they were generally in bad health, most commonly with diabetes, sclerosis of the liver, and hypertension. Gibbons tabulated all the cancer cases he and his colleagues had treated in a five-year period and found that in one area where the Navajo represented 40% of the whole population, they accounted for only 3% of the cancer cases. In another reservation, during the period 1960–73, there were only 13 cases of cancer out of 13,000 admissions. Dr Gibbons said:

> The nutritional content of their diet is a disaster. Their sanitation in many cases is unbelievably bad. Many draw water from open creeks and have no sanitary facilities (not even outhouses, much less indoor plumbing and running water). In short, they do everything wrong. And yet they do not get cancer! They must be doing something right that the rest of us are doing wrong.

Dr John Heinerman, PhD, who followed up this information in collaboration with Dr Gibbons, confirmed the generally unhealthy lifestyle of these American Indians and said:

> Many of the Havasupai menfolk smoke to some extent. Yet neither Dr Gibbons nor ourselves ever found any recorded cases of lung cancer among them. Equally amazing is the epidemic of obesity among both tribes, particularly the women. Yet no cases of breast cancer or colon cancer have ever been detected.

Dr Gibbons noticed that Navajo had a taboo against eating chicken or other birds, and wondered whether this abstinence had any connection with their freedom from cancer. This taboo aside, their current lifestyle and diet is enough to warrant a cancer incidence much the same as other Americans. Perhaps they suffer less stress, less air pollution, maybe get a little more exercise, but one thing sets them apart is the fact that they have 'no sanitary facilities, not even outhouses'. This is, perhaps, the key — the thing they are doing right that we are doing wrong — they are squatting to defecate while the rest of America is sitting on a pedestal toilet.

(A brief history of the pedestal toilet is provided as Appendix E.)

HIGH PROTEIN INTAKE

Correlations between dietary fat and cancer have been evident for many years, and similar correlations exist with high protein intake.

The optimum amount of protein for adult human consumption is about 5% of total intake. The typical Western diet based on animal flesh contains on average about 15%, as does a vegetarian diet based on grains and lentils. (It should be remembered that, cholesterol aside, vegetable protein is as potent as animal protein, and that a diet containing liberal quantities of grain products, beans and lentils will provide as much protein, or more, than a diet based on meat and poultry.)

Dr Broda Barnes of California ascribes the association of high protein diet with cancer as being due mainly to hypothyroidism brought about by the demands of protein metabolism upon the thyroid.

Cooked protein is difficult to digest and, when incompletely digested protein enters the colon, it putrefies and ammonia is formed.

On the connections between protein, ammonia and cancer, Dr Willard Visek, Professor of Clinical Sciences, University of Illinois Medical School, said:

> In the digestion of proteins, we are constantly exposed to large amounts of ammonia in our intestinal tract. Ammonia behaves like chemicals that cause cancer or promote its growth. It kills cells, it increases virus infection, it affects the rate at which cells divide, and it increases the mass of the lining of the intestines. What is intriguing is that within the colon, the incidence of cancer parallels the concentration of ammonia.

DIETARY TESTS ON ANIMALS

When dietary tests are conducted with animals, the 'test' animals are compared with 'control' animals (that is, animals on a standard diet).

In a test using the virulent carcinogen aflatoxin, rats fed a diet containing 20% protein all developed cancer, but those fed a diet containing 5% protein developed no cancer at all. A similar test in which large amounts of sugar were added to the diets of both groups was described by Dr M H Ross:

40% of the rats still alive after one year, whose intake of both milk protein and sugar was high, developed spontaneous tumours of all kinds throughout their bodies. In contrast, only 20% of the rats on low protein, high sugar intake developed tumours. Further, coronary arterial atheromatoid lesions and unusually high blood levels of cholesterol were found in rats maintained on high protein diets, even without extra fat. And after one year, 75% of the rats on high protein developed kidney disease.

MEAT

Meat is not an ideal food for human nutrition, especially cooked meat. It contributes large amounts of fat and protein and substances known to be carcinogenic, at the same time it contains no fibre and therefore causes constipation. It also contains cholesterol, which inhibits the immune system. Meat, when it is cooked, damages vital organs and undergoes chemical changes that are capable of actually causing cancer. In addition, growth hormones given to beef cattle to make them grow faster can have the same artificial stimulating effect within the body of someone who eventually eats the beef.

THE CONSUMPTION OF MEAT IS CONDUCIVE TO CANCER

Dr John Berg and associates of the US National Cancer Institute and associates at Tohoku University School of Medicine, Japan, studied 179 colon cancer patients and 357 non-cancer patients, all Japanese of varying origin and background, and found that consumption of beef was the only factor common to all the cancer patients.

A study published in the *Journal of the National Cancer Institute* in 1993 showed that men who ate the most meat had a 164% higher risk of prostate cancer than moderate meat eaters, but the greatest risk of advanced (lethal) prostate cancer was for those who ate the most fat.

Dr Raymond Shamberger of the Cleveland Clinic Foundation has identified in beef, and to a lesser degree in pork, chicken and fish, the potent carcinogen malonaldehyde. This chemical begins to form in flesh soon after death. Left-over food contains more of it than fresh. The measurement of malonaldehyde content has been used in the food industry for years to determine if food is stale or rancid, but it was not known to be carcinogenic.

Cooked meat causes damage to all vital organs, and it must be clearly understood that in order to prevent cancer or reverse it, these organs must be capable of reasonable function.

One hundred years ago, Dr Charles De Lacy Evans, who had been a surgeon in an English cancer hospital before devoting his career to natural medicine, described the cancer inducing properties of meat. He added:

'When meat is given, it should be boiled, and the liquid broth, soup or beef tea, thrown away. It contains the irritating constituents of the flesh which encourage the growth of cancer.'

DIETARY CHOLESTEROL INHIBITS THE IMMUNE SYSTEM

Dietary cholesterol specifically inhibits the anti-cancer action of macrophages, the large white cells of the body's immune system.

An animal experiment reported in *Nature* in 1978 showed that dietary cholesterol paralyses the macrophages. Two groups of animals were fed a synthetic diet containing 8.5% protein and only 1% fat, the same diet which has been shown to support healthy growth in children. Cholesterol, the equivalent of two eggs a day (600 mg) for a human, was added to the diet of the test group. Both groups were given a carcinogen to promote cancer. At the end of one year, 100% of the cholesterol group had cancer, with 90% deaths. The other group suffered only a 20% incidence of deaths from cancer, and the remaining 80% stayed perfectly healthy and free of cancer.

CHICKEN

Chicken is of course a form of meat, and like red meat its quality may vary depending on its source. Dr Virginia Livingstone, a cancer specialist of San Diego, was convinced that the consumption of chicken presented a distinct cancer risk and she believed this to be due to a microorganism commonly found in chickens that could cause cancer in people who ate chicken. This was despite the fact that she knew the same microorganism, which she called Progenitor Cryptocides, resides harmlessly in healthy humans. Her contentions were unconvincing but it is of interest to note that the feeds upon which commercially produced chickens are raised commonly contain antibiotics, growth promoters and germicides. Whether, and to what extent, this sort of chicken may contribute to the incidence of cancer is not known.

GRAIN PRODUCTS AND LENTILS

Although grains and legumes form a substantial proportion of the diets of most population groups around the world and are widely regarded as health foods, they are far from being ideal sources of nutrition. They contain large amounts of complex carbohydrate in the form of starch, which makes for great demands on the digestive system and wear and tear on the digestive organs, they contain excessive quantities of protein, and are grossly deficient in vitamins C, B and A and other important nutrients essential for the maintenance of homeostasis in the body. Apart from being acid-forming in the body, grains and legumes contain the harmful substance phytic acid which renders the minerals and nutrients calcium, iron and zinc unusable.

Processed starch food taken in large quantities is associated with stomach cancer. An Israel study described by Jane Brody and Arthur Holleb showed that stomach cancer incidence was greater among people consuming high levels of bread, noodles, cereals, beans and nuts.

A low fat, low cholesterol diet is no guarantee against cancer unless toxaemia from other sources is avoided, and such toxaemia is possible on a high protein vegetarian diet containing excessive quantities of grain products and lentils. A heavy dependence on grain products — while lowering blood cholesterol levels, improving circulation and keeping the bowel swept clean of dangerous bacteria — exacerbates arthritis and produces acid toxaemia, a chemical imbalance caused by excessive acid production.

As I mentioned earlier, my observations of conscientious followers of the Pritikin diet led me to suspect the heavy dependence on grain products, having previously noted the exacerbation of arthritis that accompanied excessive intake of these foods. (For details of the connection between excessive grain consumption and cancer, refer back to Chapter 4.)

SUGAR

In a 43-country survey by the British Cancer Institute, refined sugar featured as the primary dietary factor in breast cancer; fat was the secondary factor and protein the third.

Dr Victor Bagnall showed sugar consumption to be correlated to breast, prostatic, ovarian, bladder, intestinal and rectal cancer. Dr Joseph Issels of Germany also has made this correlation.

SALT

Salt is a powerful irritant and a strong inhibitor of enzymes, as well as interfering with circulation by causing fluid retention in the tissues. Even in small quantities, salt has been observed to increase the rate of cancer growth, an event which is not surprising in view of the fact that homeostasis within the body is entirely dependent on a proper supply of enzymes.

It is because salt is such a powerful inhibitor of enzymes that it performs so well as a food preservative. All fresh food contains enzymes which after a while will decompose it, and salt prevents this happening. Not only does the preserved food place additional demands on the digestive enzymes of the body, but salt's adverse influence is continued within the body after digestion.

Dr E D Robinson of the National Biochemical Laboratory, Mount Vernon, New York, considered common salt 'the most active cancer cause among inorganic agents'. Dr Albert Schweitzer, when he went to work in Africa in 1913, said he knew of no cancer there among tribespeople and put this down to their diet: 'The ... natives 200 miles from the coast consumed no salt. Later, when these natives started using salt, we have seen cases of cancer in growing numbers in our region ... Salt is the chemical enemy of potassium, and can cause body chemical imbalance.'

Dr Max Gerson, who claimed a 50% success rate in treating cancer patients given up as hopeless by other doctors, was more specific in his condemnation of salt. Although he accepted there were innumerable influences which combined can lead to cancer by way of slowly wearing out the liver and kidneys, he held that salt added to food was distinctly a major influence, and in *A Cancer Therapy: Results of Fifty Cases* he devoted an entire chapter to salt. Gerson's observations over many years, together with the observations of many other researchers, led him to conclude that salt was implicated in many other disease conditions, including migraine, lupus and tuberculosis.

RAW FOOD VERSUS COOKED FOOD

The main factor underlying the disease called cancer is the cooking of food — not just because of the deleterious effects on the food — but chiefly because cooking renders palatable the animal protein and fats and grains that cause most of the harm. Foods that in their natural uncooked state would be rejected by humans are made edible and tasty by cooking and flavouring.

COOKING DESTROYS NATURAL ENZYMES

As long ago as 1829, Vincent Priessnitz of Silesia discovered the adverse effects of eating cooked food. He fed two pigs on experimental diets — one on cold raw foods, the other on hot cooked foods. When he killed the pigs, he discovered that the pig fed on the raw food had firm healthy flesh but the flesh of the pig fed on cooked food was inflamed and brittle.

Not only does the cooking of any food deplete its nutritional value and tends to produce pathogenic substances, it also destroys natural enzymes which normally assist in the digestive process. Whereas a healthy person can supply from body sources the necessary enzymes in adequate amounts, regardless of whether enzymes are contained in the food or not, ailing people or the elderly may to a varying extent lack this capability. In this latter case, eating cooked food may deplete enzyme reserves to the detriment of proper metabolism elsewhere in the body.

The greatest demand on the digestive organs is the digestion of cooked food, particularly meat and cereals, and it should be remembered that the constant consumption of cooked food produces marked hypertrophy of the pancreas due to the high workload placed upon it to produce the digestive enzymes extra to normal requirements.

Dr Edward Howell of Chicago pointed out, over 40 years ago, that the hypertrophy of organs consequential to excessive function often proceeds to the atrophy of exhaustion, and that atrophy of the pancreas occurs in many terminal wasting diseases.

COOKED FOOD EXCITES THE IMMUNE SYSTEM

In addition to the depletion or destruction of enzymes, vitamins and minerals, other pathological changes occur in food when it is cooked and this is indicated by the excited reaction of the immune system when the food is eaten. According to Paul Kouchakoff, MD, of the Institute of Clinical Chemistry, Lausanne, the white blood cell count of a healthy person increases to a level proportional to the degree to which the food has been heated or processed, and may double or even treble. This effect is called 'leucocytosis'.

COOKING DEPLETES THE MINERAL CONTENT OF VEGETABLES

Probably one of the greatest drawbacks, at least in the cooking of vegetables, is that whether damaged or not, much of the mineral content is lost anyway in the cooking water when it is poured down the sink.

VITAMIN, MINERAL AND ENZYME DEFICIENCIES

Most people in Western countries, mainly by virtue of the fact that most of the food they eat is cooked or processed in some way, are likely to be marginally supplied with many vitamins and minerals. At the same time their enzyme systems will be overtaxed, often to the extent of damaging the pancreas, and it is not surprising that patients with chronic disease conditions usually display a number of deficiencies. As already mentioned, cancer patients usually display low vitality, low enzyme levels and low body temperatures.

VITAMIN DEFICIENCIES

Drs A Goth and I Littmann, in a paper entitled 'Ascorbic acid content in human cancer tissue', described how cancer most frequently originates in organs whose ascorbic acid (vitamin C) levels are below 4.5% and rarely grows in organs containing ascorbic acid above this concentration. Dr Kasper Blond was of the opinion that 'if a patient has less than 10 mg% of vitamin C in his blood one is justified in suspecting cancer'.

Due to the fact that vitamin C is so poorly provided in the Western diet, and indeed in any diet not containing great quantities of fresh raw fruit and vegetables, there is little doubt that deficiency of this vitamin is a significant factor in all forms of cancer, a point forcefully presented by Nobel Prize winner Linus Pauling and his co-author Ewan Cameron in their book *Cancer and Vitamin C*.

Other deficiencies most commonly associated with cancer are those of vitamin A and vitamin E, and many people as a protection take these substances in synthetic form.

Vitamin A supplements

The extent to which large doses of vitamins contribute to optimising blood chemistry would depend on the body's immediate requirements and the extent to which the diet is already meeting them. In some cases assistance could prove vital and in other cases, superfluous or possibly counterproductive.

In 1994 the *New England Journal of Medicine* reported a large scale trial involving almost 30,000 male smokers in Finland. Half were given large amounts of supplementary vitamin A and half were given only a placebo. The result was that those receiving the supplementary betacarotene showed at the end of the trial an 18% higher incidence of lung cancer. However, the men who at the beginning of the trial had the highest levels of betacarotene in their blood (that is, betacarotene derived from their diet) experienced the lowest incidence of cancer. Thus there is speculation about overdosing, and also the relative value of synthetic betacarotene to natural betacarotene.

The advice is to get your vitamin A from fresh fruit and vegetables because, as commented by Dr Joy Kenney, Nutrition Research Specialist at the Pritikin Longevity Centre, there may be other biochemical elements accompanying betacarotene in natural foods that play a part.

MINERAL DEFICIENCIES

Essential minerals are needed by the body to make enzymes, hormones, bone tissue, and so on. Mineral imbalance, even in an otherwise healthy diet, can severely impair the body's homeostasis, leading to symptoms of all kinds or the exacerbation of existing symptoms.

Mineral deficiencies most commonly associated with cancer are iodine, selenium, magnesium, potassium and germanium, and many people as a protection take these substances in synthetic form.

Potassium and iodine are particularly important minerals, deficiencies of which are constantly associated with cancer in many medical research papers, it being well known that cancer cells display low potassium levels and high sodium levels (salt is sodium chloride).

Dr F W Forbes Ross of England, in his book *Cancer: Its Genesis and Treatment*, emphasised the paramount importance of potassium in the diet in the prevention and reversal of cancer, and claimed that an adequate intake of potassium not only prevented cancer but allowed a high proportion of his patients to achieve complete remissions of it. He advised patients to supplement their diets with bicarbonate of potash.

It should be noted that both potassium and magnesium are poorly supplied in meat, eggs, cheese, fat, sugar and grains.

Mineral deficiencies in plants usually occur because one or more trace minerals may be lacking in the soil in which the food plant was grown. Crops which are grown in deficient soil display poor condition and are susceptible to disease and attacks by pests.

Animals are more prone to display signs of mineral deficiencies than humans because humans consume food usually imported from all over the place whereas animals graze in the same areas all the time. There are, however, some more or less isolated areas where people are dependent on crops grown in mineral-deficient soil, such as in certain areas of Europe where iodine is lacking and people therefore are prone to goitre (enlargement of the thyroid gland caused by iodine deficiency).

Andre Voison, in his book *Soil, Grass and Cancer*, demonstrated the subtleness of biochemistry. Voisin described the functions of the various trace minerals in normal metabolism and the operation of the immune system, in particular the role of magnesium, copper and zinc in the functioning of the immune system.

He also emphasised that administering mineral salts to experimental animals led to wrong conclusions being formed because the only way the body can properly assimilate minerals is in organic form, having been first taken up from the soil and changed to a colloid form by the plant used as food. The aforementioned vitamin A trial in Finland supports this contention. However, there is ample evidence that in many cases where deficiencies of vitamins and minerals exist, supplementation, properly prescribed, can provide great benefit. The evidence also shows that, to be effective, the supplements should derive from an organic source.

Minerals leach from the soil to the sea

Dr Maynard Murray,* who was convinced that faulty nutrition was the major factor in human disease, explained how over centuries minerals leached by rain from the soil end up in the sea, and that soil is made further deficient with each crop sent to market. While minerals can be replaced by using fertiliser and cropping continued, the crops will always be deficient for human use unless every one of the required minerals is present. According to Dr Murray, seawater contains all the trace minerals needed by humans. In fact, the mineral content of seawater is practically the same as blood.

In his 40 years of experiments using seawater in carefully measured amounts as fertiliser, he proved his beliefs by showing that his experimental crops produced superior growth and health in animals of all kinds.

Regarding the beneficial qualities of seawater, Dr Murray said:

> The disease resistance of plants and animals in the sea is remarkably different from disease resistance in land animals and comparisons between animals of the same or similar species are most interesting. For example, fresh-water trout all develop terminal cancer of the liver at the average age of 5½ years; cancer has never been found in sea trout. It is also known that all land animals develop arteriosclerosis, yet sea animals have never been diagnosed as arteriosclerotic. Investigators have also established the startling absence of 'chronic' disease forms, but especially the general vigorous health of sea animals that has apparently lengthened life many times in comparison to similar land species. These longevity differences are especially evident in such sea mammals as whales, seals and porpoises who have identical physiological systems with the majority of land animals important to man. And the major differences between sea and land life appear to be attributable to the superior food chain of the sea!

Dr Murray's many experiments with all kinds of crops and animals all showed dramatic benefits from sea minerals. For instance:

> Started feeding mice, both experimental and control, food that was raised on the Ray Heine and Sons Farm. The experimental food had been raised on soil fertilised with 2200 pounds (per acre) complete sea solids. The control food was the same as the experimental with the exception that it was not fertilised with complete sea solids. The food consisted of a combination of one part soybean, two parts oats, four parts corn, balanced food proteins, carbohydrates and fats for mammals.

* BSc 1934; MD 1936, University of Cincinnati; five and a half years' post-graduate study of internal medicine and ear nose and throat specialty. Taught and directed experiments at University of Cincinnati from 1937 to 1947, thereafter in private practice in Florida. Author of *Sea Energy Agriculture* and many research papers.

C3H mice [a particular strain used for experiments] were obtained for this feeding experiment. This strain of mice has been bred so all the females develop breast cancer which causes their demise. The mice were two months of age when received and started on the feeding experiments. The life expectancy of this strain for females is no more than nine months which included the production of two or three litters. The experimental and control groups both consisted of 200 C3H mice and those fed on control food were all dead within eight months seven days. The experimental mice that were fed food grown on the sea solids fertilised soil lived until they were sacrificed at 16 months; definitive examination revealed no cancerous tissue. The experimental group produced ten litters compared to the usual two to three litters and none developed breast cancer.

In the next experiments, twenty-four rabbits were obtained. Twelve were designated experimental and fed on food grown on sea solids while the remaining twelve were labelled control and fed accordingly. All of the rabbits were given a high cholesterol diet for six months which produces hardening of the arteries. The control group did develop hardening of the arteries and all had died within ten months. The experimental group did not exhibit hardening of the arteries.

And finally, on the subject of seawater minerals is an item from the *Queensland Fruit and Vegetable News* of 18 September 1986:

There may be hope forAustralian deserts if recent Israeli research is any indication. Today thirsty plants are not only drinking but thriving on seawater at an experimental farm near the town of Ashkelon on the Mediterranean Sea. Dr Dov Pasternak from the Bokyo Institute of Ben Gurion University, is overseeing the project which is studying 150 species of plants irrigated by seawater.

The research into seawater for irrigation is directly related to the successful efforts of Dr Samuel Mendlinger, also from the Bokyo Institute, to produce a special strain of sweet, high quality autumn melon growth on brackish water using drip and sprinkler irrigation.

Among other fruits and vegetables being successfully irrigated by saline water from underground aquifers are asparagus, broccoli, sorghum, olives, peas, and pomegranates.

Agricultural production in 14 southern Israel settlements is now based on underground saline water, and instead of costly desalination Israelis are taking advantage of Nature's abundance, learning to harness sea and sub-soil water to grow crops.

The best sources of minerals
Because the content of various minerals in a plant can vary enormously — depending on the soil, the water content of the soil, the weather and so on

— this means that *the best way to obtain your minerals is from a variety of fresh, raw fruits and vegetables*. Apart from vitamins and other nutrients in raw fruit and vegetables, the abundance of organic minerals they contain explains why patients with cancer respond so well when restricted to these foods.

Although organically grown fruit and vegetables are to be preferred, it should be noted that no matter how carefully organic farming is practised, the resultant crops will be lacking in quality if the soil is deficient in any one of many minerals. The produce may look good but it will lack in taste and nourishment.

People can obtain all the colloidal minerals they need by taking about a teaspoon of fresh seawater a day, according to Charles B Ahlson's *Health from the Sea and Soil* which describes the remarkable health improvements people with different ailments gained simply by taking fresh seawater. It is important that the seawater is fresh and unheated, because once heated the minerals lose their colloidal status necessary for the body to utilise them properly.

Fresh kelp and even dehydrated kelp is a good source of minerals from the sea, and it is becoming common practice for farmers desiring the best crops — while at the same time avoiding poisonous spraying — to fertilise them with fertilisers derived from sea kelp.

VEGETABLES AND HERBS

HEALTH BENEFITS OF FRESH VEGETABLES
Early in 1984 the National Cancer Institute reported a study in North Carolina which showed that women who ate less than two servings of fresh fruit or vegetables a day were three times more likely to develop cancer as women who ate four or more servings a day.

Protective enzymes
It is recognised that all the many nutrients, some of them still possibly undiscovered, play a part in the chemistry of every cell. Dr Leo Wattenberg, working at the University of Minnesota School of Medicine, discovered that rats fed a balanced, highly purified diet containing all known vitamins and nutrients were not able to make certain enzymes in the liver which inactivate cancer-causing chemicals. However, when the rats were fed a crude diet containing alfalfa (known in Australia as lucerne), they were able to produce the enzymes. And when alfalfa alone was added to the purified diet, this caused the enzyme to be made. Other experiments showed that this enzyme increased protection against cancer even when cancer-causing chemicals were added to their diet.

Dr Wattenberg found that cabbage, Brussels sprouts, turnips, broccoli, cauliflower, spinach, dill and celery also caused the enzyme to be made but varied in effectiveness according to their freshness and the soil in which they were grown.

He identified the chemicals in the vegetables which cause the protective enzymes to be formed. They belong to a well-known family of organic chemicals called 'indoles'. He also found that citrus fruits contain 'flavones', which are chemicals that have the same effect as indoles.

Dr M R Mainlow of the Oregon Primate Research Centre showed that when alfalfa was added to experimental diets it lowered the assimilation of cholesterol from food. In tests on monkeys and rabbits, assimilation was reduced from 76% to 47%.

A controversial substance

Amygdalin is a substance contained in many kinds of plants and is claimed by many people in the field of cancer treatment to be capable of inhibiting or destroying cancer cells. Amygdalin is also known as vitamin B17 or under the trademark Laetrile, and is in common use by unorthodox practitioners as a primary anti-cancer agent. The results obtained from its use have varied widely and have been inconsistent and inconclusive, and there has been great controversy in medical circles about it. It is evident, however, that when good results have been obtained using amygdalin it has always been in conjunction with modified diet usually supported by supplementary digestive enzymes, as well as in association with other lifestyle changes.

HERBS AND HERBAL EXTRACTS

There are countless herbs and herbal extracts claimed over hundreds of years in folk medicine to inhibit and sometimes cure cancer. Many of these are currently being investigated by medical researchers.

There is no question that many complete remissions of cancer have been achieved by herbal medicines taken internally and in some cases applied directly to external cancers. The famous Hoxsey Clinic in Texas successfully employed this form of treatment for many years, but although an independent investigation in 1954 by ten senior physicians from different states certified to the superiority of Dr Hoxsey's methods, the AMA eventually had his clinic closed.

Apart from inhibiting or reversing the growth of cancer, herbal mixtures have been reported to alleviate angina and reduce symptoms of diabetes, in which cases it is clear that fat metabolism and blood viscosity must be favourably influenced.

Obviously the correction of any errors, be they deficiencies or excesses, must favourably affect cellular chemistry. This may explain why, in the history of folk medicine, an enormous variety of herbal substances and extracts, used singly or in combinations, have been shown to favourably influence the course of various diseases, often effecting cures. There are far too many reports and claims of this kind, from all over the world, to be disregarded. However, what works in one case may not work in another, and with so many variables involved in the processes of cell chemistry leading to cancer, consistent results cannot be expected unless all factors are optimised.

FOOD ADDITIVES

LESS DANGEROUS THAN THE WESTERN DIET ITSELF
In July 1976, specialists from the US National Cancer Institute, American Health Federation, Harvard University, Massachusetts Institute of Technology, and the Westar Institute of Philadelphia testified before the US Senate Select Committee on Nutrition and Human Needs to the effect that the potential of food additives for causing cancer had been grossly exaggerated, but that the 'Standard American Diet' (i.e. the Western diet), high in fat, protein, highly refined carbohydrate and low in roughage, was itself the probable causative factor and certainly a predisposing one in hundreds of thousands of cancer cases each year.

LESS DANGEROUS THAN DIETARY FAT
Denmark has very strict prohibition against most food additives but has a cancer death rate 20% higher than Norway and Sweden which have far fewer restrictions on additives. Kenneth K Caroll found that the dietary fat intake per capita in Denmark was reported as 158 gm per day and in Norway and Sweden as 132 gm per day, a difference of 20%. Again the cancer rate correlates closely with the fat intake. All the observations and animal tests over and over reveal that with or without carcinogens, high fat levels constitute the greatest danger.

ALCOHOL

All alcohol is carcinogenic inasmuch as its immediate effect is to de-activate enzymes essential to oxygen respiration, and as everybody knows, its long term effect is to place excessive wear and tear on the liver. It is also a fact that while alcohol may dilate small surface blood vessels, it at the same time increases the level of blood fats thus reducing circulation and increasing blood pressure.

BEER

The consumption of beer has been associated with increased incidence of cancer of the colon and bladder. A possible link is suggested by the report from the British Regional Heart Study of 7000 men aged 40 to 60 in which it was found that heavy beer drinkers had 30% more lead in their system than light drinkers or teetotallers. Those that smoked as well had even higher levels of lead. Commercially manufactured beer also contains nitrosamines, which are carcinogenic substances.

FLUORIDE AND CHLORINE

FLUORIDE

Fluoride is an insidious, cumulative poison strongly suppressive to the immune system. It is nevertheless commonly added to water supplies as a preventative against tooth decay.

Fluoridation of the water supply is banned in Sweden, Denmark and Holland, it has been abandoned in Belgium and in West Germany, and it has never been used at all in France, Italy and Norway.

Does fluoride prevent tooth decay?

The US Centre for Disease Control and the British Ministry of Health both admit that no laboratory study has ever shown that fluoridated water is effective in reducing tooth decay. They also admit that there are no epidemiological studies on humans showing fluoridation reduces tooth decay that meet the requirements of scientific objectivity.

A study made in Holland and reported in *Science News* showed there was no reduction in dental cavities by the use of fluoride tablets or toothpaste.

What has been overlooked by fluoride supporters when they point to the significant reduction in tooth decay over the past 40 years is that the same reduction has occurred in unfluoridated areas as well.

In October 1944, the following statement was made by the American Dental Association:

> We do know that the use of drinking water containing as little as 1.2 to 3.0 parts per million of fluorine will cause such developmental disturbances in bones as osteosclerosis, spondylosis and osteopetrosis, as well as goitre, and we cannot afford to run the risk of producing such systemic disturbances in applying what is at present a doubtful procedure intended to prevent development of dental disfigurements among children ... in the light of our present knowledge or lack of knowledge of the chemistry of the subject, the potentialities for harm far outweigh those for good.

The link between fluoride and cancer

Dr J Yiamouyiannis, Science Director of the US National Health Federation, after researching the records of the National Cancer Institute covering 25 cities, concluded there is a definite link between fluoridation and the cancer death rate.

Dr Dean Burk, for 30 years in cancer research with the US National Cancer Institute and formerly Chief of Cytochemistry there, in December 1983 issued a statement of his investigations of the respective cancer death rates over the period 1940–69 in 20 large American cities, ten of which had water supplies artificially fluoridated since the mid 1950s and ten which remained unfluoridated. By 1969, the officially reported average cancer death rate in the fluoridated cities of the USA had reached a figure over 10% higher than in the unfluoridated cities. Included in Dr Burke's report was the fact that three major American courts of law had ruled that fluoridation was dangerous to health (Judge Flaherty, Pittsburg, November 1978; Judge Nierman, Illinois, February 1982; and Judge Farris, Houston, May 1982), upon which event the Chief Toxicologist of the Virginia Department of Health, Dr Brian Dementic commented: 'It appears that Drs Yiamouyiamis and Burke have correctly approached the problem and their findings stand successfully unrefuted.'

A similar correlation between fluoride and gastric cancer was reported in Japan by Drs T Okomura and T Matsuhisha, and in California by Dr Donald Austin of the Californian Tumour Registry, who reported cancer death rates in fluoridated areas to be 40% higher than elsewhere. In Canada, Dr Victor Cecilioni, comparing various Canadian cities found a similar differential of 15–20%. A general comparison of cancer death rates for 1970 of all American cities with population greater than 250,000 showed a 4% higher rate for fluoridated cities.

Fluoride is a poison

As mentioned above, fluoride is an insidious, cumulative poison strongly suppressive to the immune system. There have been a number of occasions where the concentration of fluoride in water has inadvertently reached high levels, resulting in serious sickness through poisoning. Some people have died. High levels of fluoride also cause white teeth to mottle.

Back in 1943, the *Journal of the American Medical Association* pointed out:

> Distribution of the element fluorine is so widespread throughout nature that a small intake of the element is practically unavoidable. Fluorides are general protoplasmic poisons, probably because of their capacity to modify the metabolism of cells by changing the permeability of the cell membrane and by inhibiting certain enzyme systems. The exact mechanism of such actions is

obscure. The sources of fluorine intoxication are drinking water containing one part per million or more of fluorine, fluorine insecticidal sprays on fruits and vegetables and the mining and conversion of phosphate rock to superphosphate, which is used as a fertiliser.

The journal went on to describe how further toxication was cause by fluoride emitted into the atmosphere as a result of this fertiliser manufacture as well as with the smelting of steel and aluminium, and the production of glass, enamel and bricks.

Further indictment of fluoride comes from the results of trials to ascertain whether fluoride could help to prevent osteoporosis. Quoting from *Health Freedom News*, the journal of the US National Health Federation:

> The results of these trials are now available and the conclusion is that fluoride has no place in the treatment of osteoporosis. These trials ... reported significantly increased hip fracture incidence as well as an unacceptable rate of serious gastrointestinal and osteo-articular side effects in the treated group compared with the controls.

CHLORINE

Chlorine is another chemical frequently used in water supplies. Although it is used to 'purify' water supplies, it conveys a toxic effect on those consuming the water.

Dr Edward Humphries, a veterinarian of the Bureau of Animal Health, warned in 1979 that the use of chlorine in water supplies may be lowering people's resistance to a variety of diseases. In a five-year study he noted a link between the incidence of Q fever among abattoir workers and the chlorinated water supplies in certain Australian country towns. Q fever did not appear at all among abattoir workers in towns with unchlorinated water. Dr Humphries said his study supported the research of Dr Isiah Fidler of the Cancer Research Centre, Frederick, Maryland, who found a marked depression of white blood cells in animals which drank chlorinated water.

SMOKING

A SECONDARY CAUSE OF LUNG CANCER

Smoking is erroneously held to be the prime cause of lung cancer. While smoking is a powerful *secondary* cause of lung cancer, it cannot promote lung cancer unless there first exists a pre-cancerous condition, and this fact explains the apparent mystery of why the Japanese, who smoke much more than Americans, suffer much less lung cancer. Their low fat diet protects them, as it does also against breast cancer and bowel cancer. In fact, according to Nathan Pritikin Research, in tests some years ago in Chicago in which 876 heavy smokers were checked for lung cancer, it was found that the cancer incidence was related directly with the blood cholesterol levels. The smokers with the highest levels (7.04 mm per litre or 275 mg%) had a cancer incidence seven times higher than those with medium levels, whereas there was no lung cancer at all in the subjects with cholesterol levels below 3.85 mm per litre (150 mg%).

Smoking irritates and poisons the tissues of the lungs and respiratory tract — the carcinogenic effect of which alone is capable of promoting cancer when the cancer milieu exists within the body. Deeper still is the carcinogenic effect of poisoning the entire bloodstream with various chemicals and in particular with carbon monoxide which is readily taken up by the red cells in the blood so displacing oxygen and forcing the production of extra red cells. Thus in addition to the local irritation of the respiratory tissues, not only is the liver further stressed and vitamin C destroyed, but blood sludge is increased at the same time so increasing the cancer milieu and the load on the heart.

MERCURY POISONING FROM TEETH FILLINGS

Gradual poisoning from the mercury contained in amalgam fillings has long been suspected as a cause of various chronic disease conditions.

Dr H Schwarzkopf of Germany has reported many cases in which chronically sick patients have been restored to health after having their amalgam fillings removed and replaced with gold or more recently developed inert substances. Diseases which have been reduced by this procedure, Dr Schwarzkopf reports, are cancer, erratic heart beats, pancreas weakness, erratic menstruation, headaches, thyrotoxicosis, endocarditis, hyperthyroidism, neuralgia, muscular pains and rheumatism.

Some people have found that by having their amalgam fillings removed and replaced with gold or other inert substances they have improved immensely in health.

Dental patients are not the only ones at risk. According to Dr Richard Kuninin his book *Meganutrition*, there have been numerous reported cases of central nervous system problems in dentists and dental assistants as a result of handling amalgam. Dentists have over a long period of time developed gait problems, irritability, nervousness and occasional episodes of vertigo.

MEDICAL DRUGS

All medical drugs have an adverse influence on the health of cells.

Particularly detrimental are antibiotics and chemotherapy drugs, which are by definition poisonous. They cause further damage to an already failing liver, which means they are absolutely counterproductive to the body's efforts to restore itself.

Any chemical substance taken in to the body, other than in natural form, must inevitably tend to interfere with the body's normal processes. Regardless of the short term effects, the overall effect must be to detract from homeostasis.

EFFECT ON THE IMMUNE SYSTEM

The role of medical drugs in the aetiology of cancer is probably best described in the words of Dr Harris Coulter, PhD, from his book *AIDS and Syphilis: The Hidden Link*:

> Modern scientific medical practice relies very largely on medicines whose ultimate effect is to impair the patients' immune system. This is no secret, no great discovery. It is discussed in all the relevant literature. But it has never seemed significant until today when the world is faced with an epidemic rooted in the pervasive crippling of the immune system. The drugs synthesised since the end of World War II have achieved their end — the antibiotic sterilisation, more or less, of patients' bodies — at the expense of the immune system, and AIDS is the last stop on the line. The immune system cannot be undermined indefinitely without a price being paid. The chickens have come home to roost.

Dr Robert Mendelsohn, previously chairman of the Medical Licensing Committee of the State of Illinois and Associate Professor of Preventive Medicine, University of Illinois, and author of *The Confessions of a Medical Heretic*, said:

> The next time someone points with pride to kidney transplants as being one of the greatest breakthroughs of modern medicine, you might call his attention to evidence from the Department of Surgery, University of Sydney, which shows that 44% of Australian kidney transplant patients develop cancer less than five years after surgery. A study of 400 transplant patients conducted by Dr Graham Kelly and Professor Ross Sheil pointed the finger at azathioprine and other immunosuppresive drugs needed by transplant patients as the likely cause.

It is the opinion of Dr Joan McKenna, Director of Research, T & M Associates, Berkeley, California, that the most potent factor in the destruction of the immune system, which leads to AIDS, are medical drugs, particularly antibiotics. In her research going back through old reports she found one on Pneumocystis carinii pneumonia (PCP) which is one of the classic symptoms of AIDS (immune system failure). The report concerned an epidemic of PCP after World War II, among children in European orphanages who had been given penicillin and oxytetracycline to protect them from infections. Pneumocystis carinii exists in all healthy humans and becomes pathological only when the immune system is selectively damaged. The outbreak of PCP among the orphans was not due to contagion but due to the individual damage caused to the children's immune systems by the very drugs designed to protect them.

Dr Lorne Brandes, University of Manitoba, Canada, reported links between various common medications and stimulated cancer growth in test animals. These medications included antihistamines (such as loratadine, astemizole and hydroxyzine) and antidepressant drugs (such as fluoxetine and amitriptyline).

DRUGS TO PREVENT CANCER, ACTUALLY CAUSE IT

Tamoxifen is a synthetic hormone designed to prevent breast cancer in women. A study reported by the Netherlands Cancer Institute revealed that over 25% of the women on tamoxifen developed endometrial cancer, the risk of which increased the longer the drug was taken. The same report referred to a Swedish study in which women on tamoxifen for five years had a fourfold increased risk. (Tamoxifen is also discussed in Appendix C.)

The more aggressive the drug therapy, the greater the carcinogenic effect.

The worst drugs of all to date it seems being the very drugs employed to combat existing cancer, none of which have been shown to be of the slightest assistance, while at the same time only increasing the patients' misery. (More information can be found in Appendix B.)

VACCINATIONS

It is only commonsense that foreign chemicals of any kind entering the body, particularly directly into the bloodstream, must not only tend to damage the liver but upset the body's chemical balance for an indefinite period. Dr Richard Moskowitz, of New York, in his lecture 'Immunisations: a dissenting view', said:

> Far from producing a genuine immunity, then, the vaccines may act by actually interfering with or suppressing the immune response as a whole, in much the same way that radiation, chemotherapy, and corticosteroids and other anti-inflammatory drugs do. Artificial immunisation focuses on antibody production, a

single aspect of the immune process, and disarticulates it and allows it to stand for the whole, in much the same way as chemical suppression of an elevated blood pressure is accepted as a valid substitute for a genuine cure of the patient whose blood pressure has risen. Worst of all, by making it difficult or impossible to mount a vigorous, acute response to infection, artificial immunisation substitutes for it a much weaker, chronic response with little or no tendency to heal itself spontaneously.

That the sudden introduction of a foreign substance into the tissues of the body is sensed by the body as a traumatic event is easily comprehensible, particularly when the body is that of a tiny infant, and it is little wonder that the vaccinations of infants is held to be by many doctors the prime factor in infant cot deaths. Dr Moskowitz considered all vaccinations distinctly dangerous, particularly the administration to infants of the pertussis vaccine (whooping cough vaccine), a procedure now abandoned in Germany.

What permanent damage to a tiny infant, whose immune system is still developing, could one day be displayed by illness in later life, can only be conjectured upon.

FORMALDEHYDE AND OTHER CARCINOGENS

There are innumerable chemical substances used in industry and domestically, which are known to be harmful to body chemistry to the extent of favouring the onset or growth of cancer inasmuch as when applied to animals in potent amounts in laboratory experiments they have produced cancer. Whether or not they would produce cancer in humans would depend on the extent the liver could destroy them.

Formaldehyde is a chemical used in the manufacture of many domestic products — such as particle board, insulation, plastics, disinfectants and paper products, and even toothpaste. Formaldehyde gases from these products can cause various allergic responses, such as irritation to the eyes, skin, and respiratory tract, as well as nervous disorders and asthma symptoms. In tests at the US Chemical Industry Institute of Toxicology, rats exposed to formaldehyde fumes developed nasal tumours.

THE ROLE OF STRESS

A FACTOR IN THE ONSET AND DEVELOPMENT OF CANCER
The implication of stress as a powerful factor in the onset and development of cancer has been observed by physicians for hundreds of years, it being

noted that some personalities are more prone to the effects of stress than others.

The effects of stress is to increase the level of fatty acids in the blood, increasing the blood viscosity, and to stimulate the activity of the immune system, but if the stress is prolonged and severe enough the immune system eventually becomes exhausted.

To repeat Sir Heneage Ogilvie's statement:

> The instances when the first recognisable onset of cancer has followed almost immediately on some disaster, a bereavement, the break-up of a relationship, a financial crisis, or an accident, are so numerous that they suggest that some controlling force that has hitherto kept this outbreak of cell communism in check has been removed.

A century earlier the British physician Sir James Paget wrote:

> The cases are so frequent in which deep anxiety, deferred hope and disappointment are quickly followed by the growth and increase of cancer, that we can hardly doubt that mental depression is a weighty additive to the other influences favouring the development of the cancerous constitution.

In his book *You Don't Have to Die*, Dr Harry S Hoxsey writes:

> Cancer is not only a disease, it is also a psychosis. Tell a victim he is hopeless (or let him discover it from his family) and the will to live becomes paralysed. Show him a way out, strip him of fear and hysteria, give him even a forlorn hope, and the will to live is stimulated. It becomes a powerful ally in the battle against death.

Stress is one factor in the onset of cancer. It should not be considered a cause of cancer, although it may strongly influence its progression.

STRESS OF WAR

In Chapter 8 you will read about the dramatic decrease in cancer deaths in Holland during World War II. Imagine the stress and anxiety of an entire population subjected to invasion and ruthless occupation by the Nazis for five miserable years. The cancer death rate in The Hague dropped by 30%.

World War II was also a time of sparse diets. A review of 24,546 autopsies performed in Austria revealed that in 1944, a time of great wartime stress, the death rate from heart attacks was only one-seventh of the rate in 1958 when normal peacetime food supplies were back. And that all took place before the advent of fast foods and supermarkets!

DIETARY FACTORS THAT ADVERSELY AFFECT
HOMEOSTASIS AND WELLBEING

Cancer in humans and in laboratory animals has been separately correlated in countless studies, with each of the factors listed below. Of all the influences, dietary factors are the strongest.

Dietary factors

- *Oxygen deprivation to cells*
- *Constipation*
- *High blood viscosity (sludged blood)*
- *Lipotoxaemia: high blood fat, cholesterol, various toxins*
- *Defective blood chemistry*
- *Excess body fat*
- *Excess dietary fat*
- *Excess protein (including vegetable protein)*
- *Meat eating particularly beef, smoked meat, smoked fish*
- *Dietary starch*
- *High grain consumption*
- *Salt, monosodium glutamate*
- *Highly spiced food*
- *High intake of canned, preserved or processed food*
- *Caffeine in coffee, tea, chocolate, cola drinks*
- *Cooking of food, especially fried or deep fried*
- *Low intake of fresh fruit and vegetables*
- *Vitamin, mineral and enzyme deficiencies (to a large extent caused by cooking)*
- *Fluoridated water*
- *Chlorinated water*
- *Alcohol*
- *Beer drinking as distinct from other alcohol*
- *Hormonal disturbances, particularly hypothyroidism*

ENVIRONMENTAL FACTORS THAT ADVERSELY AFFECT HOMEOSTASIS AND WELLBEING

Environmental factors

- *Hormonal disturbances, particularly hypothyroidism*
- *Lack of exercise*
- *Poor general health*
- *Stress (emotional or physical), overwork, fatigue, nagging: upsets hormonal balance, diminishes immune system.*
- *Worry, grief, despair: upsets hormonal balance, diminishes immune system*
- *Smoking*
- *Infected teeth*
- *Oral contraceptives*
- *All 'recreational' drugs*
- *All medical drugs, including vaccinations, antibiotics and, worst of all, chemotherapy*
- *Sedatives, tranquillisers, pain killers*
- *Air pollution, car exhaust fumes, etc.*
- *Various chemicals inhaled or absorbed through skin*
- *Mercury absorbed from amalgam teeth fillings*
- *X-rays, TV tube emissions, strong electrical fields*
- *Excess of sunshine*
- *Lack of sunshine*
- *Restricted circulation*
- *City life*
- *Injuries, contusions, various irritants such as asbestos particles, implants, excessively hot food: not carcinogenic in themselves, but damage sensitive tissues and promote cell division*

CHAPTER 8

Uncommon sense

*'It is the common man who keeps the wheels turning, but let us not
forget it was the uncommon man who invented the wheel.'*
— Sign outside the YMCA, Honolulu

Doctors are human, they follow their training and plod through life like
other people, some with inquiring minds and some with blinkers on.
As each generation of doctors gains experience many of them question the
value of medicine because the results they observe are so dismal. Granted,
most of their day-to-day patients survive, but usually not because of
medicine, but despite it.

You would think when even little children know that some things are
'good for you' and other things are 'bad for you', that doctors, having once
been children themselves, when confronted by a very sick patient, would
instantly inquire, 'Have you been eating anything bad for you?' But they
don't, as a rule, because their training has totally misorientated their
minds away from Nature and the fact that in Nature health is the
universal state. Like most civilised people, doctors accept disease as
simply a fairly normal part of life. But not everybody, not all doctors.

There have always been, through the generations, doctors with
inquiring minds — doctors who, when disappointed with the status quo,
look for something better. Doctors like Thomas Sydenham, William
Harvey, Richard Lambe, Russell Trall, Louis Kuhne, Charles De Lacy
Evans, Emmet Densmore, Robert Bell, Robert McCarrison, John Tilden,
Edward Howell, William Koch, Cornelius Moerman, Arbuthnot Lane,
Ferdinand Sauerbruch, Robert Mendelsohn and Max Gerson, to name a
few. There are many names, but unfortunately, not enough of them.

William Koch, Otto Warburg and Dean Burk were independent
biochemists intent on solving the problem of cancer during the early and
middle part of this century, and their conclusions were formed mainly
from observations made in the laboratory. On the other hand Robert Bell,
Max Gerson and Cornelius Moerman were practising physicians whose
observations and conclusions derived over many years of first-hand

experience with cancer patients. Their individual conclusions, arrived at by one way or another, inevitably were the same.

Long before Professor Warburg's discovery of the oxygen respiratory enzymes it had been widely known that malignancy was associated with low oxygen concentrations in the affected tissue and that cancer cells were anaerobic or partially anaerobic, being dependent on fermentation partly or wholly for their life energy just like cells in growing yeast cultures. And it was also known that cancer cells resembled the cells of a growing embryo, sometimes being indistinguishable from them, an observation that in the late 1800s led Dr John Beard, an embryologist from Scotland, to the theory that cancer originated from embryonic cells still contained in the body as undifferentiated left-overs from the embryonic stage of pre-birth growth. Beard's theory was accepted by many people for a time.

DR ROBERT BELL

Twenty years before Beard's theory was circulated, Dr Robert Bell had described how cancer cells were nothing other than cells of previously normal tissues that had undergone change and could be identified as such. As a pioneer in microphotography techniques, he had photographs of such cells.

Although there were others before him who recognised the constitutional nature of cancer and who knew that faulty diet was the underlying cause of the problem, Dr Bell was one of the first to specifically point out that cancer cells arose only in unhealthy (pre-cancerous) tissue, that they were the offspring of normal cells which had become sick, and that they were anaerobic in nature. He knew that the advent of even the smallest tumour signified not an early stage of cancer but instead, an advanced stage, stating:

> The growth, then, in its now advanced stage of its existence, being composed of cells of a fungoid nature, has ceased to conform to those physiological laws which govern normal cell life, and its characteristics have undergone a complete metamorphosis, in so far as they have become anaerobic — that is they have ceased to depend upon oxygen as their vitalising agent, and now like all fungi, absorb carbonic acid, in place of throwing it off as effete matter, which healthy cells do.
>
> Now, to understand the great change that has taken place in those cells which have undergone malignant metamorphosis, and bearing in mind that they owe their origin to normal cells, we require to note the important fact that their original and healthy condition was only compatible with their being constantly in contact

with, and bathed by, the alkaline blood, whereas when malignancy has become established, their secretions become not only highly acid, but virulently acrid, both of which features, as can readily be supposed, account for the gradually increasing rapidity of development of the tumours, which becomes more and more pronounced as time advances.

As the cancer progresses, in it can be seen the presence of degenerate leucocytes filled with innumerable spores — each of which contains a poisonous alkaloid possessing very similar properties to muscarine (the poisonous material contained in many dangerous fungi) if not identical with it.

That the fatal result, which is inevitable in cancer — unless means be adopted to check its progress — is accelerated by the toxaemia arising from the potent poison I have referred to, becomes evident, if we compare the symptoms produced in poisoning by muscarine and those consequent upon the admission of the virulent cancer juices into the circulation. These are: depression of the heart's action and respiration, destruction of the red corpuscles of the blood, increase in salivary and lachrymal secretions — all of which symptoms figure so prominently in the latter stages of the disease.

Dr Bell considered that, of all the dietary errors that together brought about the cancer milieu, the consumption of cooked animal flesh was the worst. He said:

When I was in Egypt some years ago I made the acquaintance of Professor Madden, who had given considerable attention to the subject of cancer in so far as its prevalence in Egypt, in particular, is concerned. He stated that cancer is never found in male or female amongst the black races of that country. These include the Berberenes and Sudanese, who are Mussulmans, and live almost entirely on a vegetable diet. Cancer, however, is fairly common amongst the Arabs and Copts, who form a large proportion of the population of Egypt, and who live and eat more like Europeans, thus clearly demonstrating what an important effect diet has upon this disease.

In June 1907 I received the following letter from a lady in Jersey: 'I have been so interested in reading about the cancer cure, and your views on the matter, that I cannot refrain from writing a few words which possibly may interest you. Some years ago I lived in France, where I heard cancer spoken of as *La Maladie des Anglais*. I wondered why it should be more prevalent in England than in France. I think your views about diet and attention to the cleansing of the body explain this to a great degree. Then, since I am here, I find that many Breton peasants who have left their own country to settle here, die of cancer, a disease that is unknown among the peasant class in Brittany. Probably this can be accounted for by the total changes in their food. In Brittany the quite poor, who are splendid specimens of health and strength, live on coarse brown bread and cakes of sarassin (a plant). They never touch meat, and drink cider. When they come to Jersey they work on farms, where the food consists of boiled salt pork, and vegetables, and they drink tea six or seven times a day. The teapot is always to be seen standing by the fire. A French priest told me only the other day, he could not understand why so many of his flock died of cancer.'

Dr Renner states that cancer occurs in Sierra Leone, amongst the Creoles, or descendants of liberated Africans, who have adopted the European manner of living and consume a large quantity of butchers' meat, while in the whole register there is not a single case of cancer recorded against the natives of the protectorate.

Surely these statistics will not fail to convince even the most pronounced sceptic that diet exercises a potent and unmistakable influence upon the incidence of cancer, and that the amendment of this must necessarily be regarded as an important factor, both preventative and curative.

I would draw attention to a most incontestable argument against Man indulging in the flesh of dead animals. The alimentary canal of the carnivore is short — about three times the length of the body — and the colon smooth, so that the excretions which very rapidly undergo decomposition, remain but a very short time within the canal.* Now in Man the canal is long — twelve times the length of the body — and the colon sacculated; thus unsuitable food tends to remain for a much longer period before the residue is voided. It is apparent therefore that a flesh diet is not in any way suitable to Man. Nay, more, it is not only unsuitable, but it is dangerous, and is to a large extent, accountable for the more serious diseases to which the human race is subject.

How can it be otherwise, when we know for a positive fact that uric acid is increased as much as three times above normal in flesh eaters, and the amount of urea, secreted by the kidneys, is doubled? Can we wonder then that so many people suffer from rheumatism, gout, calculus, Bright's disease and many other maladies which are distinctly traceable to this potent poison?

The viewpoint on cancer held by Dr Bell in his more mature years was, of course, entirely different from the one his initial medical training had given him. His views changed during the period in which he rose to be one of England's most eminent surgeons. By 1894 his disillusionment with the orthodox medical methods caused him to abandon surgery altogether and adopt a naturopathic approach, concentrating on patient education and prevention of disease, with the emphasis on the avoidance of toxaemia and the maintenance of a pure bloodstream.

Dr Bell used microphotography as early as 1877 to illustrate changes in blood occurring before and after the appearance of chronic diseases,

---

*Dr Bell omitted to say that carnivores consume their food raw with all its proteolytic enzymes intact to assist digestion, and that their digestive juices are, by nature, suitable for digesting meat, being extremely acid when compared to the digestive juices of humans. The human system manages by producing as much acid as it can, but this often eventually leads to stomach ulcers.

especially with rheumatism, constipation, languor, dyspepsia and ovarian disease, all of which, particularly together, indicate pre-disposition to cancer although not necessarily culminating in it.

He insisted that careful and proper attention to diet was essential, saying:

> It is essential that food should, to a large extent, consist of uncooked fruits, nuts and vegetables, and that meat be completely abstained from. Cooked vegetables or fruit should never predominate as it is essential that the vital principle and unaltered condition of the chlorophyll be retained in their natural state, and that the vegetable salts, contained in all vegetable matter, remain as Nature has provided them. Cooking has the effect of not only reducing the nutritive value of these articles but renders them more indigestible, and induces the habit of neglecting complete mastication which is an important factor in the digestive process. Moreover, the living principle, and the natural salts of fruits and vegetables are indispensable for the healthy vigour of the cells of our body, and without these it is impossible for them to retain, or regain, their physiological activity.
>
> There are three points I should insist on, viz: thorough mastication of the food so as to obtain a complete admixture of the saliva with it; a daily complete evacuation of the bowels; and living in a pure atmosphere.
>
> We perceive, therefore, that so long as the blood is maintained in a healthy condition, and the relationships of the body's cells to physiological control is thereby also maintained, healthy metabolism will continue and cancer is impossible.
>
> For really there is not a disease in existence which is, most assuredly, easier of prevention than cancer; yet there is no malady which, when once it has established its presence on a part, is so difficult to subdue.
>
> Notwithstanding that the disease has been rapidly increasing during the past fifty years until it is now 200 per cent more prevalent than it was in my youth, the public continue to cultivate it by their defiance of Nature's enactments regarding diet and hygiene.*
>
> Seneca was right when he said 'man does not die; he kills himself'. Then again it is said that 'man is as old as his arteries' when the real fact is they are just as old as he makes them.

DR MAX GERSON

Dr Albert Schweitzer said of Gerson: 'He was a medical genius who walked among us.'

---

*When Dr Bell wrote this the death rate from cancer was about one in ten. Now it is approaching one in three.

Max Gerson graduated in medicine in Germany in 1909. He practised conventional medicine but himself was plagued with migraine and could do nothing to get rid of it. That is until he started experimenting with diet. Eventually he developed a diet low in salt, protein and fat, upon which his migraine headaches no longer occurred, and so of course from that time on he treated all his migraine patients by putting them on his low salt, low protein, low fat diet, whereupon they too became free of headaches.

That this diet could allow the body to heal itself from other disease conditions was at first not apparent to Dr Gerson, but eventually this realisation occurred to him in rather a dramatic way, as S J Haught describes in his book *Has Dr Max Gerson a True Cancer Cure?*:

When the young doctor at first began to use his new therapy on his migraine patients he was jubilant to observe them all respond the same as he had done himself. But even more spectacular was his discovery when a migraine patient, whose job was in jeopardy due to his repeated absences, begged him for help. Dr Gerson noticed the man's eyelids, cheek and nose were being eaten away by disease — lupus vulgaris, tuberculosis of the skin. Nothing, he thought, could be done for that — lupus was an incurable disease — so he prescribed his diet for migraine and sent the patient home.

Not long afterwards the patient returned. 'And how is the migraine?' the doctor asked.

'Gone, all gone!' happily exclaimed the man. 'I haven't missed a day's work since!' He couldn't control his excitement. 'Doctor, do you notice anything else? My face?'

Dr Gerson leaned closer. Was it possible — the same man?

'Yes, it's true,' said the patient. 'My lupus — that horrible, ugly lupus — vanished! Like a miracle!'

It was hard to say who was the more elated — doctor or patient. Would the disfiguring scourge of lupus also respond to the migraine diet?

Before long, lupus patients were flocking to Dr Gerson's door, clamouring for the miracle they'd heard about. And wonder of wonders, the blessing repeated itself.

Other doctors, who had been echoing the ageless shibboleth of organised medicine, 'Nothing can be done,' were infuriated with Dr Gerson's success. They brought charges against him for treating skin diseases, which was not his specialty.

'I'll be very proud to be punished for curing lupus,' Dr Gerson told them. [He was prosecuted, unsuccessfully, by the German Medical Association.]

He continued to cure lupus, and by 1928 he had compiled his findings. Newspapers and magazines throughout Europe hailed the discovery, and offers from many countries descended upon the young doctor.

The bitterness of the medical fraternity knew no bounds. 'It is not scientific!' they cried.

'My answer is very short,' was Dr Gerson's reply. 'If it is not scientific to cure the incurable, then I am not scientific!'

By this time Gerson had devoted many years to his research. What a pity he had never heard of Dr Richard Lambe who in England had gone through all this one hundred years before. It is of interest to note also that Dr Louis Kuhne had employed similar dietary means to achieve exactly the same results at his clinic in Leipzig, Germany, only 30 years beforehand. I wonder if Dr Gerson had ever read Kuhne's book *The New Science of Healing*?

Lupus vulgaris is not a very pleasant sight and for that matter, not a very pleasant topic, except when you can relate of the happiness of people cured of the 'incurable' disease. Today, lupus is still considered by most doctors to be incurable.

To illustrate further the peculiar social behaviour of humans and how they unwittingly bring so much trouble upon themselves, here is a further story about lupus, taken from the autobiography of Dr Ferdinand Sauerbruch, the master surgeon who pioneered thoracic surgery and was the first to operate successfully on the human heart. Dr Sauerbruch relates:

I was sitting in a train travelling from Munich to Davos, where I had once again been invited. It had been an exhausting day and I tried to sleep, but in vain. I had probably drunk too much coffee. Grimly I leaned back and tried to read the medical journals I had with me. After we had crossed into Switzerland, another traveller got into my compartment. The man seemed bored, and it was plain that he was looking for a chance to open conversation. He irritated me by shuffling his feet, twitching his legs, fidgeting with his clothes, and by his general restlessness. Before long, he made his opening move.

'Are you going to Davos, too?'

'Yes,' I growled.

After a very short silence, he tried again. 'Are you a patient?'

'No.'

He peered across to try and read the titles of the periodicals which I had thrown down beside me on the seat.

'So you are a doctor going to Davos?'

'No, I am not.'

'Thank God for that. Doctors are fools. All but one.'

We rattled on through the night. I was desperately tired. I could not read, my eyes were aching, yet in spite of myself I was curious concerning this exception. It was not difficult to set him off again. As I stared at him, he asked, 'What can you see on my face?'

'Burns,' I suggested.

'Burns!' he cried. 'These aren't burns. They are the scars of skin tuberculosis, and I was cured of it by this doctor.'

'What!' I exclaimed, though with some restraint. Skin tuberculosis, lupus, an unsightly disease for which there was no known cure. I decided that my fellow traveller was just bragging. 'There's no cure for lupus.'

'There used to be no cure,' he replied. 'But one has been found. I have been cured.'

Before he realised what was happening, I was unfastening his jacket and shirt, for we were alone in the compartment and some distance from the next station. And on his chest I saw large areas of perfectly healed lupus. I asked him to tell me his story. From his accent, I judged him to be Russian.

The disease, he said, had developed in his home country; he had gone from doctor to doctor. Being well-to-do, he had been able to afford treatment abroad and had visited German hospitals — in vain. Feeling more and more like a medieval leper, he had been on the brink of suicide, when he was told that there was a doctor named Gerson in Bielefeld who claimed to be able to cure lupus. He decided to go to him. Why not? The effects of the disease on his face were such that he would soon be forced to retire from the world. People shrank from him, and few hotels would admit him.

As soon as Dr Gerson saw him, he exclaimed, 'Ha! Lupus, lupus vulgaris.'

'Can you help me?'

'Of course I can help you.' And he did.

I asked him how he had done so.

'By diet.'

In the whole range of medical literature, there was no reference to the treatment of lupus by diet.

'When I was cured,' he continued, 'I went to all the famous doctors who had told me there was no cure, and they all laughed at me. Doctors!'

'Did you ever go to Sauerbruch?' I asked.

'It wouldn't have been any use. He's in Munich, and anyway, he always quarrels with everybody, shouts and bellows at them. He wouldn't listen.'

I told him that I knew Sauerbruch and that I could guarantee that Sauerbruch would see him. And then he told me why he was going to Switzerland. He was hoping to acquire a building for the treatment of lupus patients free-of-charge. It was to be a gesture of gratitude for his release from this dreaded scourge. But he knew that he would need the support of some prominent man, for Dr Gerson's name was practically unknown.

'Do not forget to call on Sauerbruch,' were my parting words to him. 'I shall see that you are received by him.'

About a fortnight later, the Russian was shown into my office, accompanied by a modest man with a highly intelligent face. Dr Gerson himself, I guessed.

'So you are Sauerbruch yourself!'

Gerson declared that he had cured a number of patients by excluding salt from their diet entirely. My Russian visitor was one of them. And of his cure there could be no doubt, however amazing his claim might seem. I could see no apparent connection between treatment and cure, but that did not prevent me from beginning a series of experiments immediately.

I put my assistant, Dr Hermannsdorfer, in charge of a wing of the clinic which was fitted up as a lupus station. The patients were to be fed in accordance with Dr Gerson's diet. Lupus patients were found. We securely barred doors and windows to prevent escape. A person who, over a long period, is given food with no salt at all suffers from his situation.

Dr Gerson returned to his practice and I promised to keep him informed of our progress. Results were catastrophic. We kept the patients locked up for weeks. Not a grain of salt went into their food, but there was no trace of improvement. On the contrary, in each case, the disease advanced according to rule. Dr Hermannsdorfer and. I were at a loss, thinking of the Russian who had been cured, and of humble Dr Gerson in whom we had put complete faith.

We felt we must drop the experiment. Sadly I wrote to Dr Gerson, telling him of the failure of the experiment and our decision to close the lupus ward. I dictated that letter in the morning. That afternoon, a sister called me to an emergency case: a patient had a severe post-operative haemorrhage. I hastened along corridors and down stairs and did what was necessary. Pensively I was strolling back along the corridor near the lupus ward, when I saw a nurse, the fattest nurse in the building, carrying an enormous tray loaded with sausages, bowls of cream, and jugs of beer. It was four o'clock in the afternoon, hardly the time for such a feast in a hospital. In amazement, I stopped and asked her where on earth she was going with all that food. And then the whole story came out.

'I couldn't bear it any longer, Herr Geheimrat,' she explained. 'Those poor patients with skin TB. The stuff they are given — no one could eat it.'

She was astonished when I dashed her tray to the ground. It was one of the occasions when I completely lost my temper. Every day, at four o'clock when no one was around, she had been taking the patients a nice, appetising, well-seasoned meal.

I sent off a telegram to Dr Gerson, asking him not to open the letter I had written him. We were back at the beginning again, and from that moment we took extra precautions in guarding the lupus wing. In comparison, a prison would have been a holiday camp. Soon, Dr Gerson was proved right. Nearly all our patients recovered; their sores almost disappeared under our very eyes. In this experiment involving 450 patients, only four could not be cured by Dr Gerson's saltless diet.

Now at this time surgeons were regarded as the heroes of medicine and Dr Sauerbruch was the leading surgeon of Germany, famous in world medical circles, and he moved among the ranks of royalty and statesmen. Dr Gerson, with his now-proven track record and supported by Dr Sauerbruch, suddenly became not only 'respectable' in German medical circles but a leading figure.

In 1933 Dr Gerson was scheduled to address the Berlin Medical Association and demonstrate his cured 'incurables' (his first successes with cancer were achieved in 1928). His address was set down for 5 May 1933.

People blame Adolf Hitler and his Nazi regime for the destruction and deaths of millions of people during the days of World War II. There were other tragedies of that Nazi era, perhaps the greatest being that Dr Gerson's concepts were denied to a world ready to receive them.

In early 1933 political upheaval occurred in Germany, and Hitler and his Nazi Party took over. Max Gerson was a Jew, and in March he was forced to flee with his family to Vienna for the safety of their lives. He remained in Vienna until forced again to flee, to Paris, and then to New York, where he arrived in 1936.

In New York Dr Gerson had to start all over again. At the age of 55 he attended school with little children in order to learn English, and at the age of 57 he had to sit for all the American medical exams to gain his license to practise medicine again.

With the advent of World War II there was strong anti-German feeling in the USA, and strong opposition from the American Medical Association to unorthodox medical practice and, to make things really difficult, Dr Gerson chose cancer as his specialty. The hardest part of all was that the majority of his patients were terminal cases, given up as hopeless by the best cancer specialists in the USA. Meanwhile, back in Germany, Dr Gerson's entire family of seven brothers and sisters had been murdered in concentration camps.

Nevertheless, despite the handicaps under which he worked, and despite the fact that his patients were considered by other doctors to be as good as dead, this unflagging medical genius was able to prove a 50% recovery rate in the ranks of his cancer patients, and a success rate of almost 100% with other degenerative diseases.

In 1946 Dr Gerson became the first physician to demonstrate recovered cancer patients before a US Congressional Committee. This Senate Committee was holding hearings on a Bill to find means of curing and preventing cancer. Unfortunately, the medical lobby — supporting the orthodox treatment of cancer by surgery, radiation and chemotherapy — caused the defeat by four votes of the Senate Bill which could have supported extensive research into the Gerson therapy.

Whether motivated by professional jealousy, fear of the unknown, fear of bankruptcy or plain stupidity, the American Medical Association knowingly suppressed Max Gerson's work equally as well as Adolf Hitler and his Nazis had done unknowingly. The AMA branded Gerson a quack.

New York journalists are supposed to be hard-bitten and cynical, and when one of them — S J Haught — set out to expose Gerson as a fraud, he not only found Gerson to be genuine, but ended up writing a book eulogising him: *Has Dr Max Gerson a True Cancer Cure?*

Worn out, Dr Gerson died in 1959, of pneumonia, aged 78, just after the publication of his final work, *A Cancer Therapy: Results of Fifty Cases*, a book which provides full details of case histories, with photographs, and which should be on every doctor's desk and be compulsory reading for all medical students.

Dr Gerson, during his 50 years of constant medical practice, was the author of 55 published scientific works (and, of course, many others that were refused publication in orthodox journals).

Charitably, in the preface to his book, Dr Gerson concludes:

> The history of medicine reveals that reformers who bring new ideas into the general thinking and practice of physicians have a difficult time. Very few physicians like to change their medical approaches. The majority practise what they have learned and apply the treatments of the text-books more or less automatically. Right from the beginning, the physician wants most of all to help the patient. He hesitates to take risks for his patients by applying a non-recognised treatment. The history of science, art and technique shows that each new idea has been fought bitterly; most of the reformers did not live to see the realisation of their ideas.
>
> This is one of the reasons why developments in culture made very slow progress all through the centuries; they were restrained forcefully.
>
> I was in a more favourable position. Ninety to ninety-five per cent of my patients were far advanced (terminal) cases without any risk to take; either all recognised treatments had failed or the patients were inoperable from the beginning. It takes some time to acquire enough experience to see progress, results, or failures.

The great Dr Albert Schweitzer, concert organist, humanitarian and physician, the recipient of two Nobel Prizes, was himself freed of diabetes under Dr Gerson's care and his wife 'cured' of tuberculosis in the days when these diseases were considered incurable and fatal.

After Gerson's death Dr Schweitzer said of him:

> I see in him one of the most eminent geniuses in the history of medicine. He possessed something elemental. Out of the deepest thought about the nature of

disease and the process of healing, he came to walk along new paths with great success. He leaves a legacy which commands attention and which will assure him his due place.

THE GERSON INSTITUTE TODAY

Dr Gerson's healing mission continues today under the direction of his daughter Charlotte, who is head of the Gerson Institute in California. The Gerson Hospital and Healing Centre, CHIPSA, in Tijuana, Mexico, is operated by qualified medical doctors under Charlotte Gerson's supervision. The necessity to locate CHIPSA in Mexico is in order to avoid conflict with the US medical authorities and the Food and Drug Administration, who stipulate it is illegal to treat cancer other than by the 'approved' methods of surgery, radiation and chemotherapy.

While half a million people every year in the USA die of cancer after having suffered the approved treatments that leave many families penniless, others, fortunate enough to discover CHIPSA, fare a lot better, as this letter taken from the *Gerson Healing Newsletter* illustrates:

Dear Blanca,
Saludos.

Three years ago, having arrived three days before at CHIPSA, another tumour swiftly came up in my right axillary region. But growth stopped in three days because my immune system had kicked in. Therefore, my most exciting Tijuana experience was to see this golfball-size tumour disappear over a period of two months.

This was the last I saw of my metastatic melanoma. And here it is three years after they told me I had six months to live. I enjoy citing Psalm 30: 2, 3 (Living Bible) 'O Lord my God, I pleaded with you, and you gave me my health again. You brought me back from the brink of the grave, from death itself, and here I am alive.'

Not only am I alive but I am in top physical condition. In the last several months I've competed in the Senior Olympic Games in Michigan and Florida. I've won Silver twice and Gold once in the Racewalk. I am 67 and enjoying vibrant health. Why? Because the principles learned in the Gerson Therapy continue to apply in the maintenance of optimum health.

I teach WELLNESS both at our retirement village and in local churches. I live what I teach — I practice what I preach. To ask people to take charge of their own health and convince them that they are what they eat, is a difficult task. Even though it is dangerous to teach what the authorities say is quackery, I am committed. I feel very much like the man born blind who said to Jesus, 'One thing I do know, I was blind but now I see.'

I feel it is a privilege to be a part of the Gerson Wellness Network. As a small boy my grandfather gave me the job of watering the big draft horses. It's true —

one can lead a horse to water but we can't make them drink. I'll not tire, however, of pointing out that there is hope, even for those who've been told they are terminal.

Sincerely,
Norman R Piersma, DVM

(Further information about the Gerson's Institute's work can be found in Appendix D.)

THE UNCONVENTIONAL RESEARCH OF DR CORNELIUS MOERMAN

Dr Moerman was a university trained medical doctor and a self-trained biochemist whose determination to solve the mystery surrounding cancer began while he was a medical student in 1927.

In an examination as a student, he was asked by his examiner, Professor Tendeloo of Leyden, his opinion as to the cause of cancer. Moerman replied that he found the conventional theories unsatisfactory and said that he thought the cause of cancer could perhaps be in a local disturbance in metabolism which may have its origin in an abnormal condition of the whole body. To quote from Dr Moerman's book, *A Solution to the Cancer Problem*:

Immediately Professor Tendeloo asked: 'Can you give your reasons for this?'

I answered, 'At a lecture at the time you demonstrated a preparation that consisted of an amputated lower leg, you showed us on the leg an ulcus cruris [i.e. ulcer of the leg] that had been there for years and in which in the end a cancer had developed which had made the amputation necessary. That preparation, Professor, has still something to tell me. First of all it told me that the wound would not heal. So disease of the tissue was the primary cause. Secondarily, on this basic condition cancer had developed. Why would not the wound heal? The wounded spot was comparatively small. Also the wound was rather slight. Do you believe that this wounded spot, if it had existed in a perfectly sound organism, with a perfect metabolism, would have taken the same sad course? The healing power of a sound organism is always great enough to heal a local injury of the tissues. The local injury came from outside, but the inability to heal came from the inside. And the factor "from inside" — the disease of the tissues — I see in the first place as a *disturbance in the metabolism*. And this disturbance, if it exists long enough, might well play the principal part in the origin of cancer, irrespective of the place where the cancer appears. For here it is not a matter of ulcus cruris as such, but of the fact that it is merely an example of *tissues that are chronically ill*, which phenomenon can appear in a great number of other places in the body. This sick condition of the tissues comes first. Not until after this does cancer appear. In perfectly sound tissues cancer has never yet, to my knowledge, come into being.'

Unaware that not far away in Germany, Dr Warburg and Dr Gerson could have furnished him with a lot more of the knowledge he was seeking, in 1930 Dr Moerman commenced medical practice in Vlaardingen, Holland, determined to resolve the problem of cancer. Assistance came in from an unexpected source: he received a communication from winegrowers in which it was claimed that the number of people with cancer in the wine growing district was much lower than in places where there was little wine consumed. Moerman reflected that perhaps the citric acid and iodine contained in wine may have a favourable effect on an otherwise deficient metabolism.

His reasoning continued:

If what the wine growers had written to me was founded on truth, it was not inconceivable that ulcus cruris might be favourably influenced by citric acid and iodine. When therefore a patient came to my consulting room with an ulcus cruris that had been in existence for years, I decided not to treat this ulcus locally, but to treat the patient as a whole internally with citric acid and iodine, supplemented by a few other substances. The prescriptions I wrote were:

P. Aqua 250 gm, Citric Acid 15–20 gm a dessertspoon 3 times a day.
P. Sour red wine 300 gm, Sol. Jod. Spirit 3% 5 drops a dessertspoon 3 times a day.
P. Ascorbic acid (Vit. C) 250 mg 6 tablets 4 times a day.
P. Vitamin A 100,000 International units a day.
P. Vitamin E 10 mg 2 tablets 5 times a day.

In six weeks the ulcus cruris had completely healed. I would add that later I had to treat two more special cases of ulcus cruris, the result being the same.

Conclusion: By this means the basic condition from which cancer can develop had been conquered herewith.

People whose innovative ideas contribute to human progress do not come from a conventional mould. Dr Moerman was an unconventional doctor and his hobby was racing pigeons. Reasoning that inner body chemistry of all animals worked in the same way, biologically at the cell level, he decided to use his pigeons in his cancer experiment, and communicated with the German Bayer company who also used pigeons in experiments.

However, Moerman's approach to the problem of cancer was entirely different from that of Bayer and all the conventional researchers whose efforts to unravel the mystery were directed at producing cancer in their experimental animals and to study it from there. Instead Moerman did the opposite: he set out to find out what constituents in the diet had the effect of optimising the pigeons' health and their racing performance, which he knew demanded the maximum metabolic and aerobic efficiency which would *prevent* their getting cancer. Bayer had already informed him they could not succeed in generating cancer in healthy pigeons, which did not surprise him, but he wanted to know the dietary substances which would give them *optimum health* and render them *super-cancerproof* so that he could achieve the same results in people.

If this method succeeded, he reasoned, then he would have proven once and for all that cancer was indeed a disease of a constitutional nature, and he would have ascertained the dietary errors most commonly responsible for causing it.

The pigeon experiments that were carried out before World War II interrupted them provided Moerman with the following list of substances vital for the pigeons' best performance: iodine, citric acid, vitamin B complex, iron, sulphur, vitamin A, vitamin E, vitamin D3, to which vitamin C would have to be added because humans, unlike pigeons, cannot make vitamin C in their bodies.

Moerman found that when the pigeons were provided with adequate amounts of these substances they had healthy tissues and great vitality, whereas a depletion of the substances was followed by degeneration of the tissues and lowered vitality.

His conclusion was that humans would be affected in the same way, and that serious depletion of these same substances would lead to:

> A *sick basic condition* in which ... a local tissue defect, as for instance the ulcus cruris, cannot heal, but drags on chronically, so that embryonic regeneration cells cannot develop here into normal healthy cells, but, in a lower stage of development will make themselves *independent*, into cells with a deviating behaviour, and in this way will pass into cancer.

On the other hand, Moerman reasoned, if humans were liberally supplied with these same dietary substances they would improve their constitutional status so that no tissue anywhere in their bodies could possibly degenerate to become pre-cancerous or cancerous. It was also possible, he thought, that *cancer already established* could well be reduced or eliminated. This would be his next experiment, and one that was completely ethical because absolutely no risk was entailed. Moerman related:

> In 1939 a man came to my consulting room, Leendent Brinkman. Upon examination I diagnosed a tumour in the abdomen and a metastasis in the groin and thigh bone. Speedily I had him operated upon. The surgeon told me: 'I have operated upon Brinkman. The tumour is cancer, grown into the pelvis, great metastasis, consequently inoperable, so that I have closed the belly again without

removing the tumour. As soon as the stiches have been removed and the wound has healed, he can go home to die.'

After that I spoke to Brinkman in his house. I told him everything about my work and left in his hands the decision whether I could apply in his case the substances which I assumed to hold a possible prospect of cure.

His answer, which bears witness to wisdom and great faith, was 'Doctor, I know I am lost. But with God all things are possible. I am convinced that you will do for me everything that lies humanly in your power. Should it be of no avail to me, my body may perhaps be of some use in finding the solution ne day.'

I make no secret of the fact that these words greatly moved me.

This man was the first patient I treated with the substances I had found through experiment, combined with a diet.*

Even today he says: 'I have eaten not a wheelbarrow of oranges and lemons, but a whole wagon load.' So it is hardly necessary to remark here that I was fully conscious of the fact that in this way I had treated the man daily not with some milligrams, but with a stream of ascorbic acid so that this substance must be added to the substances found.

His reward was great. The tumour and metastases disappeared. A year later the surgeon diagnosed that he was entirely cured. Up till now, some twenty years later, Brinkman has enjoyed excellent health.

It stands to reason that this case has raised much controversy. Hardly any of the colleagues wanted to believe it. They simply said, 'It was not cancer.' When I passed it on to the Public Health Department, I was told by one of the prominent figures of the National Organisation for the Crusade Against Cancer: 'In our opinion cancer cannot be cured by medicine. If you think you have cured somebody of it, in our view it was not, therefore, cancer.'

(Dr Moerman was nevertheless lucky in his dealings with the Dutch Public Health Department; had he lived in the USA, he would have been branded a quack by the American Medical Association as was Dr Gerson. The AMA has since then lobbied to have State laws passed that make it illegal to treat cancer by any means other than surgery, radiation or chemotherapy.)

Moerman was to encounter the same obstinate rejection in the years that followed, notwithstanding the success he constantly achieved in curing many patients given up as hopeless by other doctors. Despite the clear-cut proofs he produced, none of the authoritative bodies would accept them; he said:

They would not believe me. Many prominent medical men in Holland simply said: 'That is impossible.' When I made mention of them to the Amsterdam Cancer Institute I was told by the then Director, 'If you have succeeded in discovering the cause of cancer and finding a therapy through which the morbid growth disappears, you have solved the problem. I cannot believe, however, that cancer can be cured by vitamins.'

Dr Moerman realised that the real solution to the cancer problem was not simply finding an explanation for the disease, but lay in changing people's fixed ideas, a task which could be compared to converting Moslems into Christians or vice versa. It has been a slow process, still with a long way to go.

The main thrust of Dr Moerman's argument was not to sell the idea of a 'cancer cure', but to get people to realise that cancer cannot under any circumstances arise in healthy tissue: cancer arises only in tissue which has become degenerated for one or more reasons. Direct and convincing proof of this fact has been demonstrated by Dr Gerson and a number of other researchers, and is again described by Moerman:

> If we make a burn on the back of a healthy rat or mouse, this wound will heal in the normal way. If then we subject the same rat or mouse to a prolonged action of carcinogenic substances and we make another burn [or an injury such as a cut] on its back, a violent morbid growth of real carcinoma will develop.
>
> With this we have come to the question: How must we explain this cancer growth? Cancer tissue develops on places which have suffered an injury, followed by regeneration, which means that embryonic cells are formed. And we know that the embryonic metabolism is part based on fermentation. For these cells to grow into normal cells they must be able to breathe. In a healthy body healing will follow a normal course, but will not do so in an organism where through prolonged inferior feeding the substances it needs are lacking or made inactive by carcinogenic substances which have injured the oxygenating power of the cells. The cells then will continue to ferment, they will continue on a low (anaerobic) level of development and will grow independent.

Dr Moerman then directs our attention to another experiment, one that involved the entire population of Holland and which commenced in 1940 and continued for ten years. The people of Holland were not consulted; the experiment, unplanned, was set in motion by the German occupation during World War II. As the war progressed, food became in short supply in Europe, particularly in countries largely dependent on imports from overseas. Holland was one such country in which to avoid starvation people had to rely on locally produced food. Meat and dairy products became

---

* Dr Moerman's diet was similar to the Gerson diet in which no meat, chicken or fish is permitted, nor coffee, tea or salt. Rice in the husk was permitted but the emphasis was placed on raw green vegetables, carrots, etc., as well as much fresh fruit, especially grapes. 'Orthomolecular' supplements were iron, iodine, sulphur, citric acid, and vitamins A, B complex, C and E. Later Dr Moerman added several other substances.

almost unprocurable because their production took up too much land, and people were forced to switch to a diet mainly of vegetables, and wholemeal and rye bread.

The most profound result of the change in diet was evident in The Hague, where death rates from cancer dropped sharply from a figure of 180 per 100,000 deaths to 125 per 100,000 deaths in 1945 at the war's end. In 1945 normal food supplies started to become available again. What then happened? The death ratesfrom cancer climbed upwards; by 1950 they had climbed to 160 per 100,000 deaths and have continued to rise ever since.

In regard to the list of nutrients considered especially indispensable by Dr Moerman for healthy cell metabolism, his further research indicated the importance of aneurin (thiamine, or vitamin B1), lactoflavin (riboflavin, or vitamin B2), nicotinic acid amide (nicotinamide) and pantothenic acid.

In regard to telltale signs of pre-cancer or early cancer, in addition to the signs Moerman listed from the beginning (provided here in Chapter 3, at pages 25-26), he later placed great emphasis on the appearance in the blood of virus-like microorganisms, which was the origin of the once widely held virus theory of cancer (described in Chapter 5).

As already described, the appearance of these microorganisms is a feature common to many chronic conditions, and as chronic degeneration of body chemistry is a prerequisite for cancer, many physicians, by observing the degree to which the microorganisms have proliferated, can assess the probability of impending cancer. In all cancer patients the proliferation is intense, and from this fact arose the theory that the 'virus' actually caused the cancer, a theory that has years ago been disproved.

To observe the virus, a blood sample must be examined under a microscope at the magnification of $\times 10,000$. Correct use of this method of diagnosis is far more dependable than biopsy, Moerman asserts, because it is more accurate and can be performed in a few minutes from a minute blood sample taken from anywhere in the body. Moreover, the test is much safer than a biopsy, during which there is a grave danger of cancer cells, if there are any, being liberated into the circulation to form secondary metastases elsewhere.

The presence of the so-called virus throughout the entire circulation clearly demonstrates that whatever cancer growth may be present it is a secondary effect of the primary constitutional disorder.

Like Dr Bell, Dr Gerson, Dr Koch, Dr Hoxsey, Dr Issels and many others, Dr Moerman received no cooperation or financial assistance and no recognition, from any official source, even though there was liberal granting of funds to orthodox researchers. And as with the others in his position, the majority of his patients were advanced cases pronounced hopeless by hospital specialists.

Not counting those patients with a prognosis of less than two months to live, in 1955–56 Dr Moerman treated 64 advanced cases of cancer, of which 27 people (that is, 42%) were cured, and it was his consideration that had he received an average cross-section of patients — that is, patients in the relatively initial stages of malignancy — the percentage of successes would have been much greater.

These results approximate those achieved by the abovementioned doctors, and Moerman's contention is further borne out by the claims of Drs Issels, Quigley, and Ermer shortly to be mentioned in the next chapter.

On 10 January 1987, the Dutch Ministry of Health at The Hague publicly recognised the Moerman Therapy as an effective treatment for cancer.

Dr Moerman died in August 1988, at age 95, of natural causes.

CHAPTER 9

Spontaneous remission: the reversal of the cancer process

'Our proofs stand firm, firstly in their diagnoses made by America's leading surgeons and confirmed by our foremost pathologists; secondly the cures were demonstrated to be permanent with reconstruction of tissue so good function was restored, and accomplished by a definite process without leaving even a microscopic trace of cancer cells.'

— William Koch, PhD MD, from the Foreword to *The Survival Factor in Neoplastic and Viral Disease*

Despite the entrenched belief that the only way to help someone with cancer is to either remove the growth by surgery or to destroy it with radiation or chemicals, it is common knowledge that now and again cases occur in which confirmed, well established cancer diminishes and completely disappears entirely of its own accord. This event is known as spontaneous remission, and has always mystified doctors rather than aroused their curiosity. Such is the disbelief of some doctors that they say that the patient must have been misdiagnosed, that he or she never really had cancer in the first place.

However, many cases of uncontrived, natural, spontaneous remission of cancer have been recorded. Cyril Scott, in his valuable book *Victory Over Cancer*, quotes surgeon Hastings Gilford stating in 1925:

> Though cancer is so commonly regarded as inevitably fatal, many cases are recorded of its spontaneous disappearance — and nothing can be more certain than that these recorded cases are very few in comparison with those which are unrecorded.

Dr Gilford then listed the names of many eminent surgeons and physicians who testified to their observations of spontaneous cures. Among those listed were Paget, Brodie, Muller, Sauerbruch, Gleitmann, Rohdenburg and Lomer. Lomer had recorded 213 cases of spontaneous cures and Rohdenburg 302.

Scott also quotes Dr Georgine Luden of the USA:

> The importance of this fact can hardly be overestimated. It is proof positive that the human body can wage a winning fight against malignancy under the most untoward conditions.
>
> Since outside aid had proved useless, the victory must have been won by inside means. Changes in the body chemistry, resulting from increased or renewed activity of organs by which the chemical condition in the body is regulated, seem to be the only available explanation, since the chemical composition of the blood must influence the body cells.

Now considering that these spontaneous remissions occurred 'mysteriously' and not by design, surely then with an understanding of (a) what upsets blood chemistry, and (b) what can be done to rectify blood chemistry, the chances of spontaneous remission become infinitely greater.

Sir Alexander Haddow, a medical leader in cancer research, always said the key to successful treatment lay in finding out why spontaneous remission occurred. He was not the only one who thought so, and the doctors whose stories are related in preceding chapters are ones who looked for the key and found it — to them spontaneous remission was no mystery.

CHANCES OF NATURAL REMISSION

Spontaneous reversal of the cancer process is merely a demonstration of the natural healing power of the body once it is freed of harmful influences and provided with ideal nourishment.

If proper metabolism of nutrients can be restored, auto-intoxication stopped, and at the same time the detoxifying capability of the body increased to exceed the production of toxins by the cancer cells, then favourable blood chemistry will be regained and cachexia arrested. The improved circulation and increased oxygen permeating the body acts then to retard and maybe arrest the growth of tumours and at the same time assists the immune system to regenerate. The most important factor is not the extent of the cancer, but the regenerative capacity of the body and the extent to which this can be assisted. In a critical situation it appears that the anti-tumoral effects of various herbal extracts and supplementary enzymes can be of vital assistance.

On the other hand, too rapid disintegration of cancer tissue may produce toxins faster than the body can expel them, and perhaps kill the patient. This is the reason that cancer therapists employ coffee enemas which stimulate the excretory function of the liver. It is thought that in some cases the surgical removal of an easily accessible tumour may favour the balance of factors involved.

CASES OF RECOVERIES

There have been many cases of full recovery from cancer. Most have been achieved by diet. Some have followed surgery, some have followed vitamin therapy, while others have resulted even from faith healing, meditation and various folk medicines. There are many cases of spontaneous (natural) remissions which have occurred for no apparent reason at all.

Obviously, in all of these cases, one or more of the influences we have discussed have changed sufficiently to allow the natural body functions to reverse the cancer process. There is no doubt that the faith-healing cures occurred primarily because of the patients' improved state of mind and the subsequent strengthened immune responses. The apparent medical cure could perhaps be explained by the confidence inspired by the surgeon and the relief from a stressful situation, combined with the benefits of rest and the adoption of saner living habits.

In other words, *all cures of cancer are achieved by the body itself*, when the body is given the chance to do so.

RECOVERY THROUGH DIET

The purpose of dietary correction, combined with correction of other lesser factors is purely and simply to arrange circumstances favourable for a spontaneous (natural) remission. And having achieved such a remission, and knowing how and why it occurred, there is no need to wait five years before calling it a cure, which was never more than an educated guess anyway.

Dr D T Quigley of Nebraska, an oncologist for over 30 years, has stated: 'Cancer never grows in healthy tissues but always in previously diseased tissues.' He told the American Academy of Applied Nutrition that in more than 30 years practice as an oncologist, not one of his patients who had followed his dietary recommendations had a recurrence of cancer.

Dr Walter Ermer, Executive Director of the International Health Council, reported a survey completed in 1976 on survival rates of advanced cancer patients, comparing patients on nutritional therapy with those on conventional therapy. The survey showed that patients with early or pre-cancer who adopted dietary therapy all survived, and of advanced (so-called 'terminal') cases, 86% survived, whereas of matched patients on conventional therapy only 6.4% survived.

Actress Gloria Swanson, at the age of 84 a busy sculptor and artist, described in an interview with the British magazine *Here's Health* how 50 years previously she had a tumour on an ovary which disappeared of its own accord after she gave up eating meat in 1928. She had maintained a strict natural lifestyle ever since, and said: 'You can cure anything through food. You must keep the body clean inside and it will heal anything — it repairs itself.'

There are a great number of books describing natural cancer cures, many of which have been written by medical doctors who have actually cured themselves. In her book *Cancer and Cure: A Doctor's Story*, Dr Eva Hill of New Zealand, describes how at the Hoxsey Clinic in Dallas she used methods similar to Gerson's to cure her own malignant cancer. She achieved in New Zealand similar degrees of success with patients, and of course, the same inevitable rejection by her 'peers'.

In *The Health Revolution* I described how my first wife's lifestyle led to migraine, peritonitis, asthma and heart disease and how she regained her health. What I did not mention was a skin cancer on her cheek which puffed up like a small sultana. Even though she did little exercise, the change in her diet alone was sufficient to cause the skin cancer to regress in about five weeks and completely vanish. We lived apart and I couldn't strictly supervise her diet, but it is significant that on one occasion when she felt depressed she partially abandoned the diet and I could tell simply by the reappearance of the blister-like cancer. She responded to a gentle pep-talk and again improved her diet, whereupon the cancer once again regressed and vanished in four weeks.

Actor Steve McQueen nearly made it. With only a predicted few weeks to live, he went to Mexico and undertook a dietary based 'alternative' medicine therapy for his widespread cancer. He made a steady improvement, and after three months he appeared on Mexican TV and thanked the people of Mexico for the freedom of alternative medicine doctors to practise there. As he got stronger, McQueen became impatient and decided to undergo surgery at another hospital in order to rid himself of the cancer more quickly. Unfortunately, five hours after the operation, McQueen died of heart failure caused by a blood clot from the surgery.

The case of Sir Francis Chichester
Francis Chichester's bout with cancer is a classic example of all these factors. He devotes two chapters of *The Lonely Sea and the Sky* to describing his ordeal:

> After the last sail in *Figaro*, I had a desperate attack of worry. I was
> struggling hard to make my map business pay. It was not big enough to pay
> for the new talent it needed in both the sales and the production
> department, but it was too big for me to provide all the ideas as well as the
> sales drive needed. Now I had this ghastly load of a new boat added, with
> all the extra work of planning it, and visiting it in Ireland. I had a nightmare
> fear of not being able to sell *Gipsy Moth II*, and of being landed with two

yachts. It was too much to bear. The trouble was that by the end of the Fastnet I was tired out. If only I had laid off everything for a week, I should have regained my strength to cope with things.

Cancer of the lung was diagnosed soon after this and the diagnosis confirmed by five different doctors. (Chichester was not a smoker.) He was told his only possible hope was to have one lung removed immediately. He was booked into hospital for the operation but was in such a low state that the operation was postponed. A little later he felt an irresistible urge to go to the South of France, and so went there with his wife. In 1959, in the town of Vence, he became so ill that a doctor was summoned. Chichester relates:

He examined me and said: 'Ce n'est rien, and if you follow my treatment you will be climbing up those mountains in three days' time.' The fantastic thing is that I did, in fact, climb up the Baou Blanc in five days' time. At 2200 feet it may not be much of a mountain, but it was the most wonderful climb I ever made.

What I regarded as a miraculous chain of events had started in London when I felt the urge to go to the South of France. There I reached a doctor [Dr Jean Mattei] who had been considered one of the cleverest lung physicians in Paris before he settled in Vence; also I fetched up in a town which had been considered a health resort, with a magic quality of air for lungs, since the time of the Romans. How did this thing come about? Sheila said that the doctor gave me back my confidence, that my illness was already on its last legs.

For myself, I think that some part of my body had ceased to function, that the doctor had correctly diagnosed what this was, and supplied the deficiency. To me he was a wonderful man; short, nuggetty, fit with terrific energy exuding strength and activity. He never seemed to stop work, seeing thirty patients a day at times. I heard tales of his sitting up all night with a seriously ill patient, for two nights running.

It was in April when I fell into the good doctor's hands. In June I accepted an offer to navigate *Pym* in the Cowes-Dinard race.

Of his wife, Chichester says:

She has a strange and amazing flair for health and healing. She believes most strongly in the power of prayer. When I was at my worst, she rallied many people to pray for me, my friends and others. Whether Protestants, Roman Catholics or Christian Scientists, she rallied them indefatigably to prayer. I feel shy about my troubles being imposed on others, but the power of prayer is miraculous. Hardly anyone would doubt its power for evil — for example the way Australian aborigines can will a member of their tribe to death; so why should its power for good be doubted? On the material side I believe that fasting is the strongest medicine available and that it played a very important part in my recovery. I believe that my being a vegetarian for preference helped a lot.

Unfortunately, Chichester's story has an unhappy ending. He was an intelligent, courageous man, health conscious and disciplined, but at the same time badly misinformed on matters of health.

In his book *Gipsy Moth Circles the World*, he describes his food supply for his 1966 voyage. The food was carefully selected on the basis of his diet in England. The food list is a dietary disaster. Although he described himself as a vegetarian, in fact he was not, because he ate a lot of fish, eggs, cheese and milk, along with a preponderance of refined carbohydrate in the form of sugar, chocolate, honey, syrup, marmalade, jam, sweet puddings, cakes and biscuits, honey bars, glucose tablets, liquor and soft drinks, plus canned and dried fruit. On top of all that he took large quantities of butter, oil and nuts. Ketchup, yeast and coffee were further accessories.

And although he had written a book on physical fitness, it was a subject he did not understand. His recommended exercise program does not achieve the protective 'training effect' of aerobic exercise desirable when on a diet of inferior food.

If, in addition, you add the unremitting stress to which Chichester subjected himself throughout his entire life, then it is clear that despite having achieved complete remission of his lung cancer in 1959, Chichester's mode of life and diet was one which almost guaranteed a further onset. He remained free of cancer until 1971 when it was found he had cancer of the spine. There was no recurrence however, of lung cancer.

He refused to rest — it was not in his nature — and he died, aged 70, in August 1972.

Chichester's demise was tragic; it was a case of good intentions and dedication ending in disaster because of misconceptions. His recovery from lung cancer had been assisted by fasting but he did not realise why. He placed great importance on physical fitness but did not understand the physiology involved. He felt that the prayers of his friends had assisted in his recovery but did not understand the physiology of stress.

The case of Dr Anthony Sattilaro
A happier story is that of 48-year old Dr Anthony Sattilaro, President of the Philadelphia Hospital, USA, who, like Dr Eva Hill mentioned above, achieved a complete cure. The story first appeared in the *Saturday Evening Post* in September 1980, and later in Dr Sattilaro's book *Recalled By Life*.

Full of drive, Sattilaro consistently overworked; always under pressure, he ate 'on the run' during the day and indulged in fine restaurant foods in the evening.

In May 1978 he decided to have a check-up, and the first X-ray disclosed a large tumour in his left side. A bone scan revealed cancer in his skull, right shoulder, two back bones and sternum, and a large tumour in the sixth left rib. Further tests showed cancer of the testicles and the prostate filled with it.

Although his survival chances were rated at zero, he underwent surgery and hormone treatment. His weight increased from 65 kg to 77 kg (145 lbs to 170 lbs) and his pain became so severe and constant that he was given pain medication consisting of a 'cocktail' of morphine, cocaine and compazine.

In August his father died of cancer in New Jersey. On 9 August 1978, during the drive home from the funeral, Dr Sattilaro did something that usually he would never do — he picked up two hitchhikers. This act saved his life, and indirectly, probably the lives of many others. One of the young hitchhikers went to sleep on the back seat and the other, Sean McLean, talked with Sattilaro.

As Dr Sattilaro revealed his reasons for the trip, he told his listener that he was dying of cancer.

Sean McLean replied: 'You don't have to die, cancer isn't all that hard to cure.'

Of this, Sattilaro said later: 'I looked at him and thought he was just a silly kid.'

About a week later, Sattilaro received a package in the mail from McLean. It contained a book called *A Macrobiotic Approach to Cancer*. He examined it cursorily and was about to toss it in the waste basket when he noticed a testimonial written by another Philadelphia physician who had successfully treated herself for breast cancer with macrobiotic methods.

On 24 August 1978, in a 'last-chance' attempt at survival, Sattilaro introduced himself to 30-year-old Denny Waxman, director of the Philadelphia East West Foundation, which instructs people in macrobiotic dietary principles. Waxman advised him to adopt this diet but to omit fish, oil, flour products and fruit initially. Dr Sattilaro was disbelieving, but had nowhere else to go and so embarked upon the diet.

In two weeks most of his pain had gone and he discontinued medication except for the oestrogen. He experienced a feeling of well-being which he could only ascribe to the diet, and yet his lifetime of medical training did not at first allow him to believe in it. He had one relapse of pain when he departed briefly from the diet, but thereafter has stuck strictly to it.

His weight reduced to his normal 65 kg (145 lbs) and he continued to improve.

In June 1979, after a consultation with Michio Kushi, the president of the

East West Foundation, he took himself off oestrogen and he continued to get stronger.

On 25 September 1979, he underwent an exhaustive examination in his own hospital, and the other physicians were stunned at the result. He was completely free of cancer.

Garth's story
The following letter illustrates the importance of diet in the reversal of cancer:

Dear Ross,
I know this letter will find you in the best of health. Just thought I would tell you how I am since I got rid of my bowel cancer and pancreas cancer ten years ago.

I've been very well and very active, lots of swimming and ballroom dancing. Restored 2 beautiful Jaguar cars and a couple of Harley Davidsons which I go touring with from time to time.

Over the last couple of years I relaxed a bit on my diet and started to put on some weight, in fact about 1½ stone [9.5 kg]. I began to feel a bit sluggish and without the endless energy I'd been enjoying and started getting my arthritis back in the old injuries I'd had in race falls when driving trotters years ago. I blame all the bread I'd been eating. Also noticed my bowel habits were not as good. So I decided to do something positive and went on the 'grape diet' for three weeks.

Started out with a two day cleansing fast drinking only rain water, after which I ate only grapes and drank only freshly squeezed grape juice or water. This is what happened.

Days 3, 4 and 5. Bad headache. Took long walks 2–3 miles [3–5 kilometres], 100 deep breathing and swam 200–300 metres per day in the sea. Meditated half an hour twice a day. Ballroom dancing twice a week. Plenty of rest. After day 3 had an enema daily to clean myself out. White flakes and mucous in urine.

Days 7 to 11. Felt great most of the time, occasionally felt tired, but was doing a lot of physical work.

Days 12 to 15. Didn't feel quite right but kept up program.

Days 16, 17. Bad headache, pain in colon. Still flakes and mucous in urine.

Days 18, 19. Blood in stool.

Day 20. Blood and passed what looked like a growth or polyp with mucous. Felt a bit panicky.

Day 21. Less blood in stools. Urine clearing, skin cancers on hands fell off.

Day 22. Slight trace of blood.

Day 23. No blood in stools, had a check-up with doctor. Blood pressure was 120/80, heart rate 57. Doctor took blood sample.

Day 24. Still on grape diet, no more blood in stools. Feeling of 'euphoric bliss'.

Day 25. Felt about 16 years old. Changed diet from grapes to raw juicy fruits and salads for five days, then returned to the grape diet for a further ten days. Checked weight, I'd lost the 1½ stone and was feeling fabulous.

Went back to doctor for the results of my blood tests. He said: 'Garth, I am amazed, your blood pictures are marvellous. BIZ, folic acid, cholesterol, triglycerides, sugar levels all perfect.'

I wanted to prove that the medical people have got it all wrong. When will they wake up?

Ross, during this period of time, a friend of mine was in the last days of living with his second bout of liver cancer. Some seven years ago when he was only 57 I helped him get over his first bout using the raw fruit diet. Unfortunately he got the idea later on it was OK to eat lots of pasta, spaghetti etc. and he started drinking again and let his diet go. Anyway, after seven years of good health, his liver cancer returned and his family asked me if there was anything more we could do. This was during my 'Grape Cure' so I suggested he could gain some more time and quality of life by doing the same thing. He was already bed-ridden in the Hospice.

Anyway, my friend soon made another comeback and in a few weeks was looking good, walking 3 km a day getting stronger all the time. The red blotches on his hands disappeared. I thought he had it made, but what happened then? His girlfriend, a nurse, was convinced he was not getting enough protein and urged him to eat more solid food, starting off would you believe, with a salami sandwich.

The red patches came back on his hands, he went quickly downhill and was dead in a couple of weeks. His liver was shot and he didn't give it a chance. Still after being given only three months to live in 1987 at least he got another seven good years.

The cure lies in purifying the blood and letting the liver regenerate instead of poisoning it with chemotherapy. I could tell you a dozen truths of sick people who have made fabulous recoveries using the grape diet but you can't afford to resume old bad habits.

Ross, thank you again for the books you have written, especially *The Health Revolution*, the one that got me going in 1983. You have done a fine job for humanity and I salute you. Wishing you all the best,

Yours sincerely,
Garth Squires

DR JOSEPH ISSELS

In the 1960s Dr Joseph Issels, at his Ringberg-Klinik in Germany, proved a 17% cure rate in the many 'hopeless' terminal cancer cases treated there. His story is told in Peter Newton-Fenbow's book *A Time to Heal*. Newton-Fenbow achieved a complete remission of widespread 'terminal' cancer while following Dr Issels's treatment.

Dr Issels's concept of the cancer problem is described in his own book, *Cancer: A Second Opinion*:

> The conventional idea on cancer is that it is a local disease affecting — initially — one part of the body and requiring localised therapy in the form of either surgery or radiation or chemotherapy or a combination of these. This is not my opinion. Here in the Ringberg-Klinik we believe that cancer can never occur in a healthy body ... We therefore believe that the tumour develops because of an illness of the entire body and therefore the tumour is a symptom only of the body's chronic illness.
>
> Therefore a purely localised therapy which concentrates upon the removal or destruction of the tumour itself will not be highly effective. It is also necessary to treat the entire patient.

Issels's treatment combined conventional treatment with diet, relaxation and positive thinking with which he endeavoured to restore the action of the body's immune system and general health, and he placed great importance on the removal of diseased teeth. He was emphatic that the patient should be fully informed, and said:

> In the twenty years of experience with the so-called incurable, I have seen what reservoirs of undreamed-of strength and courage can be drawn upon, even in terminal cases by the adoption of a positive attitude. I have found that a patient, previously depressed and without hope, has started to live again, provided he has had the opportunity to talk about his complaint and its implications to the doctors and his relatives.

Diet was considered important and was carefully composed with a view to wholesomeness. Here is where Issels erred badly when assessed from the Gerson viewpoint, because although the Ringberg-Klinik diet excluded ham, bacon and pork, it contained nuts, yoghurt, eggs, vegetable margarine, cheese, meat, fish and honey. Thus the worst cancer factor — lipotoxaemia — would still substantially remain, particularly when walking was only mildly encouraged. Notwithstanding these faults, he achieved comparatively excellent results. (Dr Gerson's success in achieving complete remissions of cancer was much greater because his dietary methods were much better.)

In 1969 Professor John Anderson, of Kings College Hospital in London, visited Issels's clinic and stated:

> Based on a survey of the clinic and its patients and on statistical evidence about the survival of these patients, I am of the considered opinion that this is a new approach to cancer treatment and appears to be a considerable improvement on what is usually offered ... Some of the cases I saw would have been regarded as hopeless by physicians in the United Kingdom ... the Issels' approach to the treatment of cancer is a unique and pioneering solution to a very difficult problem ... Dr Issels is an able physician, a shrewd and penetrating clinician ... there can be no doubt that he is genuine in what he does and the results he gets ... He is undoubtedly producing clinical remissions in patients who have been regarded as hopeless and left to fall back on their own resources.

Dr Denis Burkitt supported Professor Anderson's recommendation that Issels's methods be fully investigated, but the recommendations received no further support and nothing ever came of it.

Both Gerson and Issels fought against the blind rejection of the 'establishment' and were both supported by Dr Albert Schweitzer. On their last parting, Dr Schweitzer said to Issels: 'Now colleague Issels, I must return to the Wild, but you must return to the Jungle!'

THE POWER OF POSITIVE MENTAL ATTITUDE

It should be realised that for prayers to work, as in Chichester's case, it is necessary for the patient to be aware of them and so feel the encouragement and morale boosting of his friends. Chichester's reference to the bone pointing rituals of Aborigines is valid, but they too, like voodoo, only work when the victim is aware. The influence for good or evil functions by way of the subject's own mind.

Travelling by bus recently from Brisbane to Surfers' Paradise I chatted with the driver of the bus most of the way, for an hour or so. He told me of an incident he was involved in at Cairns in Queensland a few years ago to do with an Aboriginal man who was wasting away as a victim of a 'bone pointing' ritual. The Aborigine was a town dweller but still strongly influenced by tribal ceremonies and beliefs and was reduced to a dying condition.

The driver, in collaboration with some friends, contrived to perform an operation on the stricken man whereby they actually made an incision in his side, and by sleight of hand produced a piece of bone. Having convinced the Aborigine that the harmful influence was gone, the man rapidly regained good spirits and good health.

The victim in this case did not have cancer (at least not in the accepted sense) but he was being destroyed by hormonal disruption of his internal milieu just as surely.

Another example of the influence of faith is the case of former US Major-General (now Episcopal minister) John Medaris, who, at age 79, cleared his body of cancer within a few months. He said: 'People who have a positive fighting spirit and who don't give up hope stand a much better chance of fighting any disease. If you're not at peace with yourself and God, if you're mixed up inside and have inner conflict, your healing is adversely affected.'

One of Medaris's physicians, Dr James Maxfield of Dallas said: 'It's unusual for a man to have three types of cancer and open heart surgery and still be going strong. There certainly is a factor of faith in his case.'

In 1976 Dr Ian Gawler, a veterinarian from South Australia, was told by a specialist he had only two or three weeks to live. Within a few months Gawler had cleared the cancer throughout his body. The case was described by Dr Ainslie Meares in an article in the *Medical Journal of Australia*:

> This young man has shown an extraordinary will to live. He has consistently maintained a rigorous discipline of intensive meditation from one to three hours daily. He has developed a state of calm which I have rarely observed in anyone, even in oriental mystics. It would seem as if the patient has let the effects of the intense meditation enter his whole experience of life. His extraordinary low level of anxiety is obvious. It is suggested that this has enhanced the activity of his immune system by reducing his level of cortisone.

Dr Gawler said he believed the cancer was the physical manifestation of disharmony within: 'I believe that the disease is the end stage of your soul trying to tell you something is wrong.' It is interesting to note that he also incorporated strict diet in his recovery program.

Dr O C Simonton, formerly Chief of Radiation Therapy at the USAF Medical Centre at Travis Air Force Base, has used psychology successfully in slowing and arresting the growth of cancer. The first patient he treated this way was a 61-year-old man with throat cancer so severe that he could hardly swallow liquids. Dr Simonton said:

> I had him relax three times a day and mentally picture his disease. I had him visualise an army of white blood cells coming, attacking and overcoming the cancer cells. The results of the treatment were both thrilling and frightening. Within two weeks his cancer had noticeably diminished and he was rapidly gaining weight. The man had a complete remission.

Dr Simonton and his wife, Stephanie, a psychotherapist, in 1978 co-authored the book *Getting Well Again* which describes how emotional factors not only strongly influence the chances of developing cancer in the first place but just as strongly influence the chances of survival. They declared:

> You are more in charge of your life — and even the development and progress of a disease, such as cancer — than you may realise. You may actually, through a power within you, be able to decide whether you live or die.

Dr Hans Selye, the doctor who more than anyone else has drawn the world's attention to the importance of stress management, commented on the Simontons' book, saying:

> The authors appear to have caught the very essence of the stress concept, especially as it concerns the goal of overcoming cancer. Since I myself have endured and overcome an allegedly incurable cancer by means of a code of behaviour very similar to theirs, this opportunity to express my admiration for the Simontons' volume gives me great pleasure.

It should be noted that when complete remissions of cancer are achieved by psychological means, such events must be regarded only as remissions and not cures, because unless the milieu within the body has been rectified and homeostasis restored, the recurrence of cancer at some later date is always on the cards.

WARNING FROM A DANISH PHYSICIAN

In her book *My Experiences With Living Food*, Dr Kristine Nolfi reported that, having completely cleared her breast cancer by rigid dieting, the cancer re-appeared after she resumed eating small amounts of cooked food. Upon resuming her raw-food diet of vegetables and fruit her cancer again disappeared. This has happened with a number of people who have again cleared themselves by resuming the strict diet. On the other hand, others have returned to eating cooked food without trouble.

In his book *Breast Cancer: A Nutritional Approach*, Dr Carlton Fredericks says:

> Tissue which has suffered dietary insult will recover, but it remembers the transgressions. It may take five years of the average American diet to cause severe problems. Once corrected by proper diet ... it may take only two months of poor diet to awaken all the old symptoms. Under the microscope the tissues show no change, but they remember, implacably.

People who survive their first heart attack usually modify their lifestyle, at least a little, with the view of staying around as long as possible, and evidence of this is the diminished death rate by heart attack over the past 20 years since more people have learned a bit about fat and cholesterol. Smart people, of course, avoid a first heart attack altogether or at least postpone it a while. However, 'the spirit is willing but the flesh is weak', and what often happens is that, having rid themselves of their angina pains for a while, there is a common tendency for recovered patients to lapse back into old bad habits and renew old risks. This is human nature.

With cancer, as with heart disease (they often occur together anyway), the stakes are the same — your life — but with cancer the chances are more slender, for several reasons:

1. People, including doctors, know much less about what causes cancer than they know about the causes of heart disease, which means that little effective advice for prevention or cure is available.
2. While cancer cannot kill as suddenly as a heart attack or stroke, by the time it is usually discovered the internal damage to vital organs is greater, so that far sterner measures are required to reverse it. It is easier to clear blocking arteries by diet than it is to clear a malignant growth.

Nevertheless, there is more than ample evidence to show that the best chance of recovery from cancer lies in working for a natural spontaneous remission. Having achieved a total clearance of cancer, however, it must be taken into account that one or more vital organs may not have regained full function and that to remain permanently cancer-free, great care should be taken to maintain homeostasis within.

CONCLUSION

Now that the physiological effects of diet, physical exercise, stress, rest, sunlight and so on are more fully understood, they can now be properly considered as interrelated instead of separate factors. Particularly with cancer, every single component involved must be corrected simultaneously to ensure best results.

It is clear that spontaneous remission of cancer is best achieved by attending to every detail, correcting every one of many possible factors, but it cannot be over-emphasised that by far the two most important factors are a strict and uncompromising adherence to a natural diet and a powerful will to survive.

CHAPTER 10

Dieting for health and longevity

'The Art of Living consists of dying young, but as late as possible.'
— Anon

Dieting for health and dieting for longevity are not necessarily the same thing. Whereas dieting for immediate health improvement is of course worthwhile, a diet which may accomplish this in the short term may not necessarily be good enough to get the best long term results. Dieting for longevity therefore must not only provide all the body's present requirements for good health, but do so with the least amount of strain on the vital organs in order to avoid as long as possible the degeneration we call 'old age'.

The health of the body is only as good as the health, collectively, of all the body's individual cells. In turn, the health of the cells is determined by the quality of the lymph fluid that bathes them (that is, the *milieu interieur*), which again is dependent on the purity of the bloodstream. Toxaemia is the enemy.

So while it has long been a medical dictum that 'a man is as old as his arteries', it is equally true that 'a man is as healthy as his blood'.

The composition of the blood is very complex and is maintained by the combined actions of all the vital organs. From the point of view of nutrition, it is the liver which takes in the products of digested food and redistributes them into the bloodstream to suit the rest of the body's requirements. And it is the liver and kidneys which receive back, also by way of the blood, the waste products of all the cells from which they sort out what components can be used again and what must be thrown out in the urine. For the maintenance of correct blood sugar levels, the liver depends on information from the pancreas, a dual purpose organ which not only secretes the insulin and glycogen used in the control of blood sugar but secretes, as an entirely separate function, the primary digestive enzyme juices used in the digestion of food. In the beginning and in the end, the status of health is determined almost entirely by the quality of the diet, because it is from the materials available in the diet that the liver constructs and orchestrates the entire spectrum of chemical processes upon which life depends. The design of the system is perfect — it is the quality of the diet that lets it down.

THE NATURAL DIET OF HUMANS

Towards the end of World War II, when the Americans invaded the Philippines and recaptured them from the Japanese, a lone Japanese soldier ran off into the jungle there and hid, firmly believing that sooner or later the tide of battle would turn again and Japan would in the end be victorious. He decided to wait things out in the jungle. He waited 25 years, all the while avoiding human contact, and then one day emerged from the jungle and surrendered.

Upon his return to Japan he was medically examined. The soldier amazed everybody — he looked so young compared to other middle-aged Japanese men. His teeth were perfect and his eyesight too. He displayed none of the usual signs of degenerative disease considered normal in civilisation. And yet his life had not been easy.

The only possible explanation for his physical preservation was that his diet for 25 years had been fruit, berries and various plants eaten raw — a diet similar to that of wild primates and that of early humans before the domestic use of fire.

HOW OUR DIET EVOLVED

Life of all kinds is most prolific in tropical regions both on land and sea, and this is not to be wondered at because it is in warm and moist conditions that enzymes work most efficiently. In such a warm, moist environment it is thought that life first appeared on Earth, and it is generally accepted that it was in the tropical regions that the early primates evolved from lower forms of life, to be followed by the evolution of the apes and then by the first humans.

In the plant kingdom, fruit trees were late arrivals on the evolutionary scene and it is highly probable that fruit-bearing trees and primates evolved concurrently, which accounts for the development in the primates of stereoscopic colour vision, grasping hands, specialised teeth and jaw structure, appetite for sweet tasting food, medium length digestive tract, and so on. In their symbiotic relationship, the fruit trees provided the primates with food and the primates unknowingly spread the fruit seeds wherever they ate or defecated, so ensuring the continued survival of the trees.

The study of comparative anatomy and the different natural diets of animals in the wild indicates strongly that the natural diet of early humans consisted predominantly of sweet fruits, and that even though millions of years have passed, the basic anatomy and digestive apparatus of humans have not changed and are therefore still best suited to fruit as the most suitable food. That this opinion is not just idle speculation can be quickly proven by any sick person who can break the addiction to our modern taste-stimulating foods and go on a diet of good quality fruit for just a few days. Of course the human digestive system is quite capable of handling foods of animal origin, including animal fats, but in only very limited amounts can it do so without strain, even when the foods are eaten raw as intended by Nature.

Thus it can be surmised that the ideal diet for humans is one mainly of sweet fruits supplemented by various berries, green nuts, shoots and occasionally small amounts of foods of animal origin, all eaten raw. This is the sort of food eaten by our closest relatives in Nature, the orang-utan and chimpanzee, both of which have an anatomy and digestive system almost identical to ours. Neither of these animals in the wild display tooth decay or any of the other diseases common to humans, but soon do so if kept in captivity and fed cooked and processed food.

WHY OUR DIET CHANGED

There is not a population group anywhere today who, as a general rule, eats uncooked natural food: the majority of the world's populations base their diets on cooked grains of some kind or other, and the rest base theirs on cooked animal products supplemented by grain, dairy products and vegetables, all cooked. Fruit is looked upon more as a mere accessory to the various traditional diets rather than a sustaining food. How and why did this change come about?

Early humans

Early humans lived in small groups and, before the use of fire, ate their food raw like all the other creatures on Earth have done since life first began. Their senses of sight, smell and taste indicated to them the foods most suitable to their systems. Population numbers were restricted by the amount of food available growing wild. With the domestic use of fire it was found that various foods consumed by other animals, but which were distasteful to the human palate, could be made more edible by cooking, and made more tasteful by artificially flavouring them with herbs and salt. By the use of these new sources of food, greater populations could be supported, not only in areas already occupied, but in territory where food naturally suited for humans was not available.

As population pressures forced some people to move into less hospitable territory outside the tropical regions, these people of necessity became reliant on a different diet, and on fire and primitive clothing for warmth. Sickness, when it occurred, was thought to be the work of evil spirits, and so witchdoctors had to be invented.

The development of agriculture

Greater challenges in a less benevolent environment led to continued brain development, and it was in the temperate climatic zones of the world that technology commenced, leading to the advent of farming and the development of cereal crops from wild grasses. Continued competition for territory made warfare inevitable and this led again to greater technological development and so on. From all these changes a new breed of human developed — one who had become 'civilised' and had left his natural environment forever.

Next to the domestic use of fire, the development of grain crops was the greatest factor leading to the human population explosion of today. Grain could be produced easily, and being storable, provided food for all seasons. More and more forest land was destroyed to grow crops and to make pasture to raise cattle. According to their circumstances, some populations came to base their diets on meat and dairy products and others based theirs on rice or wheat or other sorts of grain.

THE PRICE OF DEVIATING FROM A NATURAL DIET

A diet based meat and dairy products does not provide ideal nutrition, nor does one based on rice or wheat or other sorts of grain.

As civilisation 'progresses' and food becomes more and more preserved, processed, cooked, and generally less and less natural, so humans everywhere display more signs of disease earlier and earlier in life.

Long ago medicine men protected us from evil spirits and disease; today the superstition of medicine has got out of hand — 'scientific medicine' has become a powerful industry consuming a vast amount of the national economy.

While the wild animals remain sleek and healthy without medicine, humans spend more and more money on 'health care' and all the while just get sicker and sicker.

The pitfalls of the Western diet are many, but it is a fact that few populations elsewhere on different diets do much better. This is because the majority of other population groups are too heavily dependent on grains of some kind as the staple of their diets, and grains are even less suitable to the human system than flesh foods.

So illness can be seen to be a human phenomenon for which there are two main causes: (a) the use of unsuitable foods; and (b) the cooking habit, necessary to render unsuitable foods edible.

THE PROS AND CONS OF COOKING

All that cooking is good for is that it enables people to utilise grains for food and it renders edible other unsuitable foods such as meat and potatoes. Thus cooking enables a lot of people to sustain themselves on the only foods available to them, but in return there is a penalty to pay.

Reference has already been made to the problems encountered by eating cooked food. And the subject has been explained in depth in two of my previous books, *The Health Revolution* and *Improving on Pritikin*. In brief, the natural digestive processes utilises enzymes existing in raw food which, when the food is eaten, perform a considerable amount of predigestion (breaking down the food) in the upper cardiac section of the stomach before the main digestive system gets to work on it. Thus a great load is relieved from the pancreas, the organ that produces the main supply of digestive juices.

This natural benefit is entirely missing when cooked food is consumed, because cooking destroys enzymes and, not only that, the pancreas is doubly penalised because of the difficult nature of the sort of food anyway when compared to the natural food the human system is designed for. Thus, as described by Dr Edward Howell in his books *The Status of Food Enzymes in Digestion and Metabolism* and *Enzyme Nutrition*, the human pancreas is invariably hypertrophied and twice its proper size compared with the relative sizes of those in wild animals and is accompanied by changes in the gonads, adrenals, pituitary and other ductless glands.

Another adverse effect of cooking is that it renders minerals in the food less assimilable, and when cooking water is poured down the sink some of the minerals are lost altogether.

Dr Max Garten, in his book *The Health Secrets of a Naturopathic Doctor*, described how his health had not much improved by becoming a vegetarian; and how this led him to try a completely raw food regime. He said:

> The results were electrifying; within a few days I felt much stronger with a return of my former enthusiasm. Many of my patients whom I had been able to convert to this new diet also reported similar results.

Dr Garten observed that putrefactive bacteria in the colon increased (and therefore the odoriferousness of the stool) not only with the eating of meat but also with the degree of heat used in cooking *all* food, and with this increase came the appearance of aches and pains. He said:

> It could only be deduced that certain agents in the diet were either missing or had been altered by the heat.

The respective protein content of the vegetarian diet had also been found to be indicative of changes in the intestinal flora, legumes such as beans, lentils, peas etc. equally contributing to the display of putrefactive changes.

Thus, although vegetarians are usually healthier and outline meat eaters, they may not maintain very good health or live to a very advanced age if they continually cook their food.

THE VERDICT

There is an association between the cooking and processing of food and the incidence of all diseases, including cancer. And, as proven in the sanatoriums around the world, the best recoveries from chronic, so-called 'incurable diseases' are made on diets composed of raw fruits and vegetables. This shows that, when vital organs are at their lowest stage of function, only such a diet makes it possible for the vital organs to provide the proper body chemistry to maintain health. That being the case, so must raw food provide the maximum benefit to anybody whether sick or well.

RAW FRUIT, OUR NATURAL FOOD

People become vegetarians to improve their health and extend their lives. Some vegetarians go a step further and consume their food mainly uncooked, while others go even further and limit their diet to fruit, which they claim to be the natural food of humans. (Remember, the requirements for protein and fat are much lower than generally believed.)

Fruit can provide the full complement of all required nutrients in adequate quantities, provided a reasonable variety of fruit is eaten. Therefore, instead of being considered merely an accessory to conventional meals, fruit should be considered in its own right as a staple food.

ADVANTAGES OF A FRUITARIAN DIET

The advantages of a fruitarian diet are many:
- It provides complete nourishment with the minimum of extraneous substances capable of 'silting' up the tissues.
- It is most easily digested, minimising the energy required for digestion (which is substantial) thereby minimising total food (calorie) requirements.
- It is palatable
- It is easily obtained and easily prepared.
- It satisfies the appetite when sufficient has been eaten — fruitarians are always lean.

- It provides minimum but adequate protein.
- It provides minimum but adequate essential fats.
- Maximum energyis available from the amounts eaten, with only carbon dioxide and water, which are entirely non-toxic, as the by-products.
- It provides the body with adequate amounts of pure water.
- It results in a favourable alkaline internal state.
- Favourable intestinal flora predominate in the bowel.
- No constipation occurs.
- No auto-intoxication occurs.
- The body de-toxifies itself.
- The blood is clean and low viscosity, there is good circulation with low blood pressure.
- There is the least wear and tear and the least 'silting up' of all the body organs and tissues.

MAHATMA GANDHI, CONVERT TO FRUITARIANISM

The Indian philosopher and statesman Mahatma Gandhi, in his book
The Health Guide, *spoke of the advantages of a fruitarian diet.*

After experiencing poor health throughout his youth, he became a student of Nature Cure at the age of 32. First he became a vegetarian and then a fruitarian. After six months as a fruitarian, he said:

'… during this period, I have been able to keep well where others have been attacked by disease, and my physical as well as mental powers are now greater than before. I may not be able to lift heavy loads, but I can do hard labour for a much longer time without fatigue. I can also do more mental work, and with better persistence and resoluteness. I have tried a fruit diet on many sickly people, invariably with great advantage. My own experience, as well as my study of the subject, has confirmed me in the conviction that a fruit diet is the best one for us.'

EVIDENCE THAT FRUIT IS OUR NATURAL FOOD

That fruit, alone, can ideally sustain human health and vigour, even without drinking water, indicates that it indeed provides the basis of the natural diet of humans. Further substantiation of this view is that there are many distinct anatomical, physiological and biological features of humans which show unquestionably that the human body is designed mainly for a fruit diet. These features include: natural fondness for sweet foods; jaw and teeth structure; salivary secretion; length of digestive tract; and size of pancreas. In fact in all these respects, humans are practically identical today with the other higher primates in the wild which, whenever possible, live mainly on fruit.

Evidence of the suitability of fruit as a staple food and not just as an accessory to the conventional diet, is to be seen by observing fruitarians who live entirely on a wide variety of fresh fruit, and who display lean, youthful bodies, low blood pressure, clear vision and unimpaired faculties, even with advancing years.

Vitamin C is not manufactured in our bodies
Further evidence that the human diet should be based mainly on fresh fruit is provided by the fact that all primates, including humans, are incapable of making vitamin C in their bodies whereas other animals can (with the exception of guinea pigs and fruit-eating bats).

This is not some 'error of Nature' — some unfavourable mutation in our evolutionary past some millions of years ago as some people contend — as the following reasons show:

1. The only mutations which persist to become a universal feature of a species are favourable ones. Unfavourable mutations cannot possibly do so.
2. A genetic change preventing the synthesis of vitamin C in the body, to become universal to an entire species, must therefore have been, at the time, a favourable change.
3. The only possibility of such a genetic change being favourable is for the species to have been already getting more than adequate vitamin C, and that any more was superfluous.
4. The only source of 'excess' vitamin C in nature is a diet of raw fruit. (Only certain tropical fruits contain such high levels of vitamin C; many fruits contain only small amounts.)

Therefore it is clear that the human diet ideally, should be based mainly on fresh fruit, and that past errors which have led to widespread vitamin C deficiencies are dietary — not genetic — errors.

The importance of fructose and the danger of sucrose
Another important food component provided by fruit (and honey), a deficiency of which is no doubt as serious as a deficiency of vitamin C, is fructose, without which the body is entirely dependent on glucose for its blood sugar.

Although fruit contains both glucose and fructose, glucose requires the presence of the hormone insulin before the cells of the body can use it to produce energy, whereas the cells can utilise fructose without insulin and thus relieve the insulin-producing cells of the pancreas of a great amount of work.

Nature provides humans with an appetite for sweet tasting food. In the modern diet the appetite for sweetness is satisfied mainly by sucrose (refined sugar), rather than by fruit. In the modern diet most of the blood sugar will therefore consist of glucose obtained from sucrose and from the conversion by the liver of other (non sweet) foods, and both these methods require considerable digestive effort.

Now while it is true that sucrose is made up of both fructose and glucose, and that the sugars in fruit are also fructose and glucose, there is a tremendous difference which renders sucrose harmful and fruit desirable.

Sucrose is not a natural substance. It is harmful because fructose and glucose — the two simple sugars of which sucrose is composed — are linked together in a chemical bond in which the body is unable to use them, so the digestive system has to separate them. This separation is accomplished by the digestive enzyme sucrase, which the body has to especially manufacture for the purpose. However, when the separation is accomplished, the effect of the enzyme is somehow to cause a rapid entry of the sugars into the bloodstream so that the blood sugar level rises abnormally, stimulating the release of insulin from the pancreas. This causes distressing fluctuations capable of producing hypoglycaemia and an increase in blood triglycerides, sometimes accompanied by various emotional problems.

The entry into the bloodstream of glucose and fructose from fruit presents no problem; the two are already separate and no enzymes are required, the glucose enters more steadily and is followed up by the fructose, which is released at a slower rate so that the blood sugar level remains steady, thus further avoiding unnecessary work by the pancreas. Although great benefits are obtainable by the substitution of sucrose by fructose in pure extracted form, the benefits fall far short of those available free from a fruit based diet. Ripe fruit and honey are the only natural sources of fructose.

Whereas most people know that vitamin C can be obtained and added to the diet if necessary to correct body chemistry, it is less well known that fructose in pure extracted form can be obtained and substituted for sucrose (refined sugar) with very favourable results. According to Professor J Daniel Palm of St Olaf College, Minnesota, some of the benefits he and Dr David Hawkins (the Medical Director of the North Nassau Medical Centre) have observed from this use of fructose are: a decrease in premenstrual tension, reduction of schizophrenia and other psychiatric disorders including hyperkinetic syndrome in children, elimination of migraine, less tendency to alcoholism and overeating, and the normalisation of diabetic symptoms.

The best fruit

Obviously some fruits are more nutritious than others, and quality will vary according to the quality of the soil in which they are grown. Commercially grown fruit may contain various levels of insecticide poisons, in which case the fruit should be carefully washed or peeled.

At the time of writing, I have subsisted almost entirely on commercially grown fruit for 14 years, all the while working long hours under stress seven days a week, and have maintained excellent health. I only eat fruit that is ripe and sweet, and I choose the fruit at random, with a preference for tropical fruits, and include dried fruits from time to time without any attempt at being scientific about it.

At my yearly pilot medical checkups, I enjoy being told by my doctor I have the arteries and blood pressure of a schoolboy. That makes fruit taste better still, even on a winter's day.

Addressing objections to fruitarian diets
Increases triglycerides?
It is claimed by some people that a fruitarian diet will eventuate in high blood triglycerides and this is why Nathan Pritikin limited fruit. The increase in triglycerides is supposed to follow elevated levels of blood sugar after eating fruit, but this does not occur with eating whole raw fruit, particularly eaten at whim throughout the day rather than in three large meals.

Erodes tooth enamel?
An objection to acid fruits such as citrus and pineapples, particularly if unripe, is that eaten in excess, the acid is said to cause erosion in the enamel of the teeth. I have not found this. It is interesting to note here that with good body chemistry and a clean mouth, teeth are more resistant to damage, and like bones are to a great extent self-repairable.

Causes digestive upsets?
It is probably best not to mix the acid fruits with others eaten at the same time. Some people find they experience digestive upsets when at first they embark on a fruitarian diet. This may be because of mixing incompatible fruits or possibly not chewing them properly. The fruit should

be taken as snacks throughout the day, as frequently as desired, rather than conventionally as three substantial meals.

If cooked food is eaten at the same time as fruit, the fruit should be eaten first as it digests quickly and clears out of the way of the other food which may reside in the stomach for several hours.

NATURAL, HUNZA AND WESTERN DIETS COMPARED

The table provides an estimated comparison of a natural raw fruit diet (such as the one eaten by the Japanese soldier mentioned earlier) with the Hunza diet and the Western diet.

The percentages given in the table are the percentages of total kilojoules (calories). Western diet contains almost double the kilojoules of the Hunza diet because the Western diet contains four times as much fat and twice as much protein as the Hunza diet. If we compare the Hunza diet with the natural diet it is clear that, notwithstanding the Hunzas' physical excellence when compared to ours, they still could have done a lot better!

DIETING FOR HEALTH

Dieting for better health has little to do with taking vitamins and minerals and eating 'health foods'. Most of the malnutrition suffered in civilisation eventuates not because of diet contains deficiencies but because it is improperly constituted.

In dieting for health it is necessary to eliminate or drastically curtail from our menus the sort of foods that cause toxaemia and lead to ill-health. This means denying ourselves a certain amount of pleasure in eating, a denial a lot of people refuse to accept on the grounds that they are not overweight and that they have 'never had a day's sickness in their life'. 'Moderation in all things' is another reason to fall back on. (Moderation, however, depends on just how long you want to last.)

Because the Western diet contains adequate quantities of all the nutrients needed to sustain life, it is considered to be 'balanced' and capable of maintaining good health. This is true only to a point: reasonable health can be maintained on the Western diet only as long as the digestive system, liver and other vital organs are capable of enduring the load the diet puts upon them as they struggle to provide a pure and complete bloodstream from processed and semi-artificial food.

STEP ONE: CUT OUT THE HARMFUL THINGS

The first thing to do in dieting for health is to cut out the harmful things. Great improvements in health can be even achieved without making any changes in the diet other than simply eating less and cutting out salt.

COMPARISON (ESTIMATED) OF THE NATURAL DIET WITH THE HUNZA DIET AND THE WESTERN DIET			
FACTOR	*NATURAL DIET*	*HUNZA DIET*	*WESTERN DIET*
Food	All raw	Some raw, some cooked	Mostly cooked
Calories for adult male (approx.)	2000	1925	3500
Vitamin C (approx.)	3000–9000 mg	adequate	100 mg
Other vitamins and minerals	adequate	adequate	borderline
Natural enzymes	ideal	adequate	almost nil
Protein % (approx.)	4% (ideal)	10% (excessive)	15% (hazardous)
Fat % (approx.)	4% (ideal)	17% (excessive)	40% (dangerous)
Natural carbohydrate % (approx.)	92% (ideal)	73%	5% (inadequate)
Refined carbohydrate % (approx.)	nil	little	40% (dangerous)
Cholesterol	almost nil	low	400 mg (dangerous)
Fibre	adequate	adequate	inadequate
Salt and condiments	nil	low	hazardous
Caffeine in tea, coffee, soft drinks	nil	low	hazardous

Drastically reduce dietary fat

Toxaemia is the enemy of the bloodstream, and lipotoxaemia ('lipo' means fat) is the arch-enemy of health. The worst feature of the Western diet is all the fat in it, and therefore regardless of anything else, our main objective must be to drastically reduce the intake of fat.

By virtue of unsticking the blood and improving its circulation and oxygen content, great benefits are felt within three or four days. With less impedance to the digestion by fat, putrefaction in the colon is reduced and therefore toxaemia from that source is reduced too. As fat severely inhibits the function of the immune system, reduction of fat brings about vastly improved immune function, also within a few days.

Regardless of which 'health diet' a person chooses, be it the European grape diet, the Pritikin diet, the Gerson diet, the Macrobiotic diet, the fruit juice diet, or just plain fasting, in all cases a great improvement in wellbeing is experienced in three or four days, the improvement being due to the fact that all these diets are very low in fat.

Medical authorities, slowly getting the message, currently recommend people should reduce the amount of fat in their diet to less than 30% of their daily kilojoule intake. This is nowhere near good enough. Some benefit is felt at 20% but for good effect the maximum should be 10%.

There are several methods of reducing fat and cholesterol in the blood. Physical endurance (aerobic) exercise produces what is called the 'training effect' by which the body becomes capable of more efficiently metabolising blood fats for the production of energy. Athletes in training therefore display lower blood viscosity, lower blood pressure, higher oxygen levels, better immune function and better general health when on the conventional Western diet than do untrained people on the same diet.

Another way of coping better with high levels of dietary fat (can you guess?) is to eat the fat raw the way the traditional Eskimos do, and allow the adipose lipase (enzyme) in the fat itself to pre-digest the fat to allow its more thorough break-down during digestion. Not that the Western diet ever contained much whale blubber, but at least once upon a time the milk, butter and cheese was unpasteurised and contained valuable enzymes.

I guess the easiest way to eliminate fat from the bloodstream is simply not to eat it in the first place, remembering that all foods contain some, the bad items being foods of animal origin, including dairy products, and of course all extracted vegetable oils and anything containing them. Animal fat of course contains lots of cholesterol too, so eliminating this fat from the diet serves a double purpose.

The body makes its own fat out of protein and carbohydrates and when refined carbohydrates, sugar and alcohol are taken, these too will elevate the amount of fat (triglycerides) in the blood.

Reduce protein

The next step in dietary improvement of course is to reduce the amount of protein in the diet. Cutting out foods of animal origin — meat, chicken, eggs and dairy products — will achieve this because these foods are the major source of protein in the conventional diet, and by eliminating them you eliminate in one move, not only excess protein but cholesterol and excess fat as well.

Conventional nutritionists usually advise vegetarians to maintain their protein intake levels by using nuts, lentils and beans (which are high in vegetable protein), but there is absolutely no need for this as our aim is to reduce protein to between 5% and 10% of our daily kilojoule intake. On a typical vegetarian diet it is difficult to get protein down to 10% anyhow.

By reducing the worst ingredients of the Western diet — excess fat, excess protein, cholesterol and salt — to safe levels, you will have eliminated to a great extent the factors underlying most of the diseases of modern civilisation, particularly atherosclerosis (heart disease), kidney disease and cancer, but it should be pointed out that the substitution of the dangerous fat and cholesterol foods with a lot of grain products can lead to toxaemia of a different kind, possibly as harmful as existed beforehand.

Cut out salt

As explained in Chapter 7, salt is a powerful irritant and a strong inhibitor of enzymes, as well as interfering with circulation by causing fluid retention in the tissues. Even in small quantities, salt has been observed to increase the rate of cancer growth, an event which is not surprising in view of the fact that homeostasis within the body is entirely dependent on a proper supply of enzymes.

Cut out (or at least reduce) grain products

Grain products (cereals) have been hailed as a health food by 'victims' of the Western diet because they are low in fat, contain no cholesterol, are high in complex carbohydrate (starch) and high in fibre the constipation fixer. Thus switching to grains from the Western diet produces immediate benefits, but other problems soon arise.

Grain products, supplying mainly starch, place a great burden on the digestive system. Mature grains contain enzyme inhibitors which prevent digestion. Grains (such as sweet corn) are digestible only if they are unripe, or if they are cooked or if they have germinated.

Even when they are cooked, the complex carbohydrate requires great digestive effort to break down, and this is demonstrated by the fact that people who consume large amounts of grains develop a pancreas double its normal size and other signs of strain such as stunted intestinal villi.

Unless rice and other grains are accompanied by liberal amounts of fresh vegetables and fruit in the diet, nutritional deficiencies occur, as well as toxaemia and acidosis capable of producing skin problems, arthritis, hardened arteries and cancer.

GETTING THE BEST RESULTS

Reference back to previous pages will remind you that a lot more improvements can still be made if you are looking for the very best results, because the question comes in two parts: (a) what immediate degree of health do I want, and (b) how long do I want it to last?

A moderate dietary change may restore a 40-year-old to good health, whereas the same change may not get the desired results in a person of 60 whose vital organs are in worse condition. The 40-year-old, as he gets older, may find he needs to be stricter with his diet to maintain good health.

A lot of people claim they don't need to diet for health at all, because they have never had a day's sickness in their life. The trouble is they cannot see the degeneration going on inside them and they don't even feel it until perhaps one day they start getting chest pains, or feel a strange lump inside them, or spit out some blood. Thus someone, proud of their vigorous health, may suddenly overnight become a permanent invalid or even be finished for good.

It is human nature to seek pleasure and to put other things aside until forced to attend to them and for this reason most people only start thinking of their health when it starts to fail. Then they want a 'quick fix' so they can return to their indulgences again. When they find medicine is a waste of time and money they may decide to try a diet. There are many diets to choose from. All of them require self-discipline because to some extent or other the seductive flavours of the Western diet must be abandoned. We are addicted to these flavours, and giving them up is as hard as giving up any other drug.

FAD DIETS
Fad diets for slimming

Although being overweight is associated with increased risk of disease and shortened lifespan, it does not follow that dieting for weight loss and dieting for health are the same. Whereas proper dieting will achieve both weight adjustment and good health together, there are some slimming diets that achieve weight loss at the expense of health.

High protein diets, for example, are effective in reducing weight but are dangerous over a period. They work because they cut down (correctly) on fat and refined carbohydrate but make the mistake of substituting high protein foods as 'filler-uppers', so increasing the intake of protein from a barely tolerable level to an even less tolerable level certain to worsen toxaemia and increase the risk of kidney failure and cancer.

Fad diets for health

In Europe the grape diet has for years been popular in various spas and sanatoriums, where sick people go to spend some weeks to recover their failing health. In a short while invalids feel great, lose weight, and so on, and then return home to indulge in their favourite foods again, planning on another spa holiday next year.

Other people go on fruit-juice fasts or grapefruit diets and get the same wonderful results while they remain away from Western style food. They almost always return to their old eating habits, not because they cannot break the habit but because they cannot break the addiction. Habit and addiction are not the same thing.

In the mid–1800s a wonderful health diet was invented by Dr J H Salisbury of New York. It was of course called the 'Salisbury diet' and so incredibly good were the results gained by it that people travelled even from Europe to be treated by Dr Salisbury. The story of the Salisbury diet is told in *How Nature Cures*, a book written almost one hundred years ago by Dr Emmet Densmore of England. I was astonished to read that the diet consisted of nothing other than lean, partially cooked ground beefsteak taken three times a day preceded an hour beforehand by a pint of hot water and another pint of water taken before retiring at night. On this diet the patients all suffered a constant craving for something sweet, but all rapidly improved in health. Although potentially dangerous in the long term, the diet achieved marvellous short term results simply because it was low in fat and devoid of starch, starch being from Dr Densmore's experience the worst dietary factor of all. In effect, the diet was equivalent to a partial fast; his patients from the Continent could have saved themselves a long trip, and achieved better results, by going to Germany and eating grapes.

FASTING

For people in well enough condition to undertake a fast, this is probably the most rapid and effective way to detoxify the body and return it to full function and health. For best results the fast should continue until the body is completely detoxified and this may take anything from a week or two to several months, depending on the individual case. Fasting must be carefully supervised and is outside the scope of this book. It is not recommended for cancer patients.

HEALTH DIETS ASSESSED FOR PERMANENT ADOPTION
The Weight Watchers diet
This diet is calculated more to achieve weight loss than to improve health but, if followed properly, both weight loss and improved health will follow. The Weight Watchers diet could be described as 'the Western diet in moderation', and health improvement can be expected mainly as a result of eating fewer calories rather than changing the kind of food. The diet is nowhere near ideal because it still permits too much protein, fat, mayonnaise, cheese, eggs, salt and pepper. But it is better than the conventional Western diet and is a good start in the right direction.

Vegetarian diet
A true vegetarian diet, which permits no foods of animal origin at all, is known as a vegan diet. A diet that permits no animal flesh nor any fish, but which includes milk and cheese and eggs, is referred to as a lacto-ovo vegetarian diet.

The obvious advantage of vegetarianism is the absence in the diet of animal protein, animal fat and cholesterol. Lacto-ovo vegetarians still take in these harmful substances because dairy products and eggs are high in them, and so they gain only partial benefit.

As a rule, most vegetarians consume a fair amount of grain products, lentils and beans and as a result still take in too much protein as well as too much starch. These foods are of very dubious value although they are widely accepted as 'health foods'. In addition, further harm ensues when vegetable oils are freely used, and when the vegetarian food is cooked — particularly if overcooked, salted and spiced.

Thus many vegetarians are not much better off, healthwise, than those consuming the traditional diet. However, notwithstanding these mistakes, the advantages of following the vegetarian way of life are still considerable, as demonstrated by statistics of death rates taken from Dr Jeremiah Stamler's lecture on a study conducted by Loma Linda University, California, on Seventh Day Adventists (discussed in Chapters 4 and 7).

The Macrobiotic diet
Any diet that drastically cuts out fat and cholesterol must, like the Salisbury diet, show good results for at least a while. The Macrobiotic diet, of Japanese origin, endows great health benefits when it is adopted by people who have been on the Western diet. The diet is based on grain products, principally brown rice steamed or boiled, which accounts for around 50% of the total intake, about 25% cooked vegetables, 10% beans or lentils, 5% miso, 5% seaweed and only 5–10% raw vegetables. Fruit is not recommended and salt is allowed.

The Macrobiotic diet is claimed to be a healthy diet and indeed, by comparison to the Western diet, may appear to be so. The diet's shortcomings are that it relies too heavily on rice and permits too much cooking and salt. As mentioned already, grains are acid-forming and heavy dependency on them can lead to arthritis and cancer.

The Pritikin diet

Nathan Pritikin claimed his diet to be the 'healthiest diet in the world'. If he was comparing the Pritikin diet to the traditional diets of the major population groups around the world, his claim would have been substantially correct. There is no question of the Pritikin diet's superiority over the Western diet for a start, and its emphasis on complex carbohydrates and reduction of protein and fat make it theoretically a far better diet than the traditional, so-called balanced diet espoused by today's nutritional experts.

The Pritikin diet achieves rapid, often spectacular results, first and foremost because of its very low fat content. It achieves reversal of atherosclerosis because of its low cholesterol content. It achieves reduction of blood pressure by virtue of unsticking the blood and lowering its viscosity, and by the same means permits the body's insulin to work better, so reversing diabetes. Lots of other good things happen simply because of improved circulation and more oxygen in the tissues.

The diet's shortcomings are that it relies too heavily on grains and permits too much cooking. As mentioned already, grains are acid-forming and heavy dependency on them can lead to arthritis and cancer.

The Gerson diet

Originally devised to solve the problem of migraine, the Gerson diet was found to be effective in arresting other metabolic and degenerative diseases, and has been used with high levels of success in the treatment of cancer since the 1930s.

The diet forbids salt and is very low in fat, cholesterol and protein. It consists mainly of raw vegetables and fruit, and juices made from these. Some cooked vegetables and rice are permitted but the diet does not contain much grains, and it therefore must be considered superior to the Pritikin diet. The results demonstrated by Dr Gerson, and later by his daughter Charlotte, clearly demonstrate this superiority.

The Hunza diet

As was discussed in Chapter 1, Major-General Sir Robert McCarrison proved that the unsurpassed health and physical endurance of the legendary Hunzas was directly attributable to the their diet.

The Hunza diet was similar to the Pritikin diet in that it contained a fair amount of wholegrain foods mainly in the form of wheatmeal bread, hardly any meat or fish, and a lot of vegetables, boiled and raw. However, the diet also contained liberal quantities of raw fruit, raw milk and cheese. There were no chickens, eggs, tea, sugar, salt or rice.

In the nine years he spent among the Hunzas, Dr McCarrison's medical skills were almost entirely confined to the treatment of accidental lesions, operations for granular eyelids, and the removal of senile cataracts, as other health problems were practically unknown. Dr Wrench, in his account of McCarrison's work, remarked upon the amount of raw food consumed by the Hunzas and attributed this mainly to be why they were so free of disease.

The raw food diet

Nobody can claim to have invented the raw food diet — it is the diet provided by Mother Nature in the first place. Dr Richard Lambe of England extolled the virtues of the raw vegetarian diet back in 1809 and described the successful use of it in the treatment of cancer patients.

Diets made up of raw fruits and/or raw vegetables have been the key to the success of famous sanatoriums in Europe, USA, Australia and elsewhere for many years. These include the Battle Creek Sanatorium started by Dr Harvey Kellogg of the USA a hundred years ago, the Bircher Benner Sanatorium in Switzerland, the Hopewood Health Centre in Australia, Dr Ann Wigmore's Hippocrates Health Centres in the USA, and more recently the Hippocrates Centre on the Gold Coast in Queensland.

The advantages of eating food uncooked are many, and result in health benefits unobtainable from cooked food. Some foods, such as cereals and potatoes, are indigestible uncooked but, as such foods are of dubious value anyway, are better left alone.

The fruitarian diet

A diet composed of high quality, ripe, raw, sweet fruits provides the human body with all the nutrients it needs with the very least expenditure of digestive effort, at the same time producing no toxic by-products, so allowing the body to detoxify itself and perform at its peak.

Raw fruits are more palatable and provide more energy for a given amount than vegetables, and can be prepared with less effort and less waste.

Not only can the highest level of health be attained on a fruitarian diet, but because it places so much less wear and tear on the body's vital organs, degeneration is slowed down and the lifespan extended.

THE FACTS AND FALLACIES OF 'HEALTH FOODS'

When you walk into a health food store and look around, what do you see? One wall of shelves is packed with vitamins and mineral products, all expensive and all unnecessary for people on a reasonable diet. Another section displays jars of seaweed extracts, sea-salt, vegetable salts, lecithin granules and so on, all of which have dubious value.

Seaweed undoubtedly contains minerals that may be insufficiently supplied in some people's diet, but sea-salt — apart from the fact it contains iodine, an essential trace mineral missing from the soil in a few areas of the world — is still plain sodium chloride (common salt), which is a dangerous product. Vegetable salt is a flavouring powder made from vegetable extracts but has little flavour of its own and so when you read the label on the jar it usually reveals the fact that ordinary salt or sea-salt forms part of the mixture.

Then you see nuts of all kinds, dried lentils, soya beans — bins full of them — foods which contain high levels of fat and protein and are stressful to the digestive system. Shelves are stacked with bottles of polyunsaturated vegetable oils — 100% fat — which although containing no cholesterol as do animal fats, nevertheless cause red cell and platelet aggregation in the blood and are associated with increased risk of cancer.

Cookies, biscuits, energy bars, some of them high in fat and sugar, none of them as healthful as a good banana. Bins of brown rice and other grains — fair enough foods if eaten sparingly — and bins of dried fruits. Dried fruits, if they are sun-dried and unsulphured, are good foods but are very concentrated and better eaten sparingly as snacks when fresh fruit is not available.

One food item which could be considered as a health promoting food is garlic, not because it provides valuable nutrients the body needs, but because of its therapeutic medicinal property in a body handicapped by a high fat diet. Garlic, onions and other herbal extracts such as vitamin E, have the effect of unsticking the blood to permit improved circulation. Used for this purpose these products are more medicines than foods, but at least garlic tastes good.

The contents of health food stores can be considered health-giving only to the extent they are less harmful than meat, chicken and dairy products. The only foods that qualify to be called 'health foods', using the true meaning of the word 'health', are fresh fruits and vegetables — you can maintain good health indefinitely on these, but the same cannot be said for the general run of foods available in health food stores.

SUMMARISING HEALTH DIETS

Leaving aside the fact that in general the cooking of food leads to an overworked digestive system and increased toxaemia, the single common denominator possessed by all effective health diets, cooked or raw, is the drastic lowering of the fat content, which allows the bloodstream to clear itself of fat and allows the red blood cells and blood platelets to unstick, so reducing the blood viscosity and permitting the blood's free circulation and oxygen-carrying ability. The enormous improvement in wellbeing that results from this single factor of improved blood condition has little to do with anything contained in the diet — the benefit stems from what has been removed.

So great is the improvement of health and wellbeing achieved by the simple expedient of improving the circulation that the beneficiaries think they have struck the jackpot; they think they have discovered the perfect diet, be it the grape diet, the Macrobiotic diet, the Pritikin diet, the Gerson diet or maybe even the Salisbury diet. And this is easy to understand, but there is more to good health than just improving the blood circulation. What about the delicate chemistry of the blood? What about the avoidance of toxaemia? The wear and tear on our internal organs? The wastage of digestive energy and valuable enzymes?

Insidious degeneration can continue undetected in a body apparently brimming with vigorous health. Probably the best example of this is the common occurrence of sudden death by heart attack of extremely fit athletes and runners who eat a high cholesterol diet. Right up until their sudden collapse, which usually occurs during or just after vigorous activity, these people display all the signs of good health. Their blood viscosity is low, because they can metabolise fat quickly from their blood, and so their blood pressure is good; they feel good, because their blood contains plenty of oxygen; they don't 'catch' colds, because their immune systems are performing properly. They are healthy in this sense, but when death overtakes them autopsies reveal coronary arteries blocked with cholesterol. They had been under the illusion that endurance exercise prevents heart disease; but the evidence is now clear that physical training does not prevent the accumulation of dietary cholesterol in the arteries, it merely maintains a better blood flow and prevents the usual symptoms of heart disease from being displayed.

Nathan Pritikin was the first one to loudly warn the public of the dangerous illusion that athletes could indulge in a high cholesterol diet and get away with it. But there are other illusions of which Pritikin was not aware. Avoiding heart disease is not the be-all and end-all in the quest for good health.

Clean arteries and thin blood are the prime essentials, and these are easily accomplished on the Pritikin diet, but they are not enough. The next step is attending to the actual chemistry of the blood and how perfect chemistry can be achieved with the least wear and tear on the vital organs.

This involves further investigation into nutrition and the enzymes that make improved nutrition possible. The subject becomes a little different from that of dieting for immediate health benefits, it becomes one of gaining long term benefits — that is, *dieting for longevity*.

DIETING FOR LONGEVITY

Do tissues and organs wear out or are they gradually destroyed by processes which could possibly be avoided?

Scientific opinion agrees that the human lifespan potential is about 120 years and some estimates go higher. These estimates are probably conservative because quite a number of people are known to have exceeded 110 years without making any special efforts at all to preserve themselves. Be that as it may, the consensus of opinion is that by taking reasonable care, the degeneration which constitutes the aging process can be slowed down so that old age is postponed.

What is 'old age'?

I would define 'old age' as a degenerative condition of the entire body, the progress of which is determined more by the degenerating factors in a person's lifestyle than by their chronological age.

Everyone knows what old age looks like from the outside, but what changes occur inside the body? In his book *The Span of Life*, Dr William Malisoff describes the atrophy and degeneration of every organ and tissue in the body that accompanies old age and the malfunctions which occur as a result. He says:

> The system of organs is so thoroughly connected that all these changes have mutual repercussions. Thus too the liver, pancreas, spleen, kidneys, urinary organs, become atrophied, hardened and degenerated. The capsule of the kidney is thickened, the parenchyma hardened; the connective tissue scleroses and compresses tubules and glomeruli, impairing their action. The changes in the brain, in the spinal cord, in the nerves, are of a similar character.
>
> The description of the changes would fill many volumes. We can summarise that they fall into several classes: the atrophies, which have been commented on; the fibroses as replacements by fibre; pigmentations; metaplasias; hyperkeratoses, or skin changes and the like; renunciation of functions, as those of the germ cells and the instance of fat cells which no longer store fat.

Dr Arnold Lorand of Austria, in his book *Old Age Deferred*, described old age as a condition in which there is a diminution of metabolism (the assimilation and conversion of food into energy), and is characterised by the abundant growth of connective tissue in vital organs, diminution of oxidation and increased auto-intoxication.

Dr Charles De Lacy Evans, in his book *How to Prolong Life: An Enquiry into the Cause of Old Age and Natural Death* written one hundred years ago, was more specific:

> The most marked feature in old age is that fibrinous, gelatinous and earthy deposit has taken place in the system; the latter being chiefly of phosphate and carbonate of lime, with small quantities of sulphate of lime, magnesia and traces of other earths.

He added that the deposits occur in all tissues including the bones and blood vessels, which harden and reduce in calibre, and quoted a Dr C J B Williams who said:

> The process is, therefore, to be viewed as almost entirely of a chemical nature, and as consisting of the concretion and accumulation of calcareous salts, phosphate and carbonate of lime in the debris of animal matter.

Dr De Lacy Evans went on to explain how the fibrinous, gelatinous substances were formed by the oxidation within the bloodstream and tissues of excessive albumin (protein), and how the earthy deposits were derived mainly from grain products, and root and leafy vegetables and to a lesser extent from animal products. Dr Evans tended to blame the formation of the fibrinous, gelatinous substances on the presence of oxygen, just as some biochemists do today with their 'free-radical' theory of aging. More pertinent to the argument, in my opinion, is that if the diet is correct then neither the excess albumin nor the free-radicals will present themselves in the first place to use the body's valuable oxygen improperly.

Dr Arthur C Giese, Professor of Biology Emeritus, Stanford University, in his book *Living with our Sun's Ultraviolet Rays*, says:

> In our multi-cellular bodies some cells, such as those of the epidermal basal layer, continue to divide throughout life; others — for example nerve and muscle cells — differentiate and cease dividing at birth. Nevertheless, they continue to function for a lifetime, with gradually lessening activity and progressively filling with insoluble wastes and pigments.

As the tissues slowly acquire these characteristics of old-age their decline is further characterised by, and is measurable by, a corresponding decrease in enzyme levels and activity. On the other hand, animal tissue cells grown in cultures in the laboratory, properly cleansed and drained, do not degenerate in this fashion and may outlast the animal from which they originated many times over. It is held by some researchers (at least in theory) that in ideal circumstances immortality is possible. Other experiments with live animals fed on minimum rations showed improved health and a life extension of 50–100% over that of unrestricted control animals on the same diet.

THOSE WHO EAT SPARINGLY LIVE LONGER: THE EVIDENCE

The longest-lived populations in the world are accepted generally to be the people of Hunza in northern Pakistan, Vilcabamba in Ecuador, and Georgia in Russia. An analysis of these people's living habits carried out under the auspices of the *National Geographic* in 1973 by Dr Alexander Leaf of New York provided a good reason why they outlived people of the Western world. The traditional diets of these long-lived (by our standards) people contained only half to two-thirds the calories of the average American intake, about a quarter the amount of fat, and half the protein. Their carbohydrate intake was about the same but was unprocessed instead of processed. As well, these people got more outdoor exercise and were less subject to stress than Americans.

Dr De Lacy Evans, when reviewing a study of centenarians in England in the 19th century, said:

> On reviewing nearly 2,000 reported cases of persons who lived more than a century, we generally find some peculiarity of diet or habits to account for their alleged longevity; we find some were living amongst all the luxuries life could afford, others in the most abject poverty — begging their bread; some were samples of symmetry and physique, others cripples; some drank large quantities of water, others little; some were total abstainers from alcoholic drinks, other drunkards; some smoked tobacco, others did not; some lived entirely on vegetables, others to a great extent on animal foods; some led active lives, others sedentary; some worked with their brain, others with their hands; some ate only one meal a day, others four or five; some few ate large quantities of food, others a small amount; in fact, we notice great divergence both in habits and diet, but in those cases where we have been able to obtain a reliable account of the diet, we find one great cause which accounts for the majority of cases of longevity, moderation in the quantity of food.

Thus perhaps the first rule in dieting for longevity is to eat sparingly, whatever the make-up of the diet. Even on a bad diet this rule will still permit better health and extended life because less wear and tear will have to be endured by the body.

So it becomes clear that 'old age' occurs because we take into our bodies harmful substances that overtax the digestive system, cause toxaemia of the *milieu interieur*, overtax the eliminatory organs, and gradually accumulate in the tissues and cells to increasingly impede their functions.

It follows then that old-age can be deferred by selecting foods that provide the best nutrition with the least digestive effort and the least amount of harmful residues, and consuming such foods in moderation.

SUMMARIZING ON LONGEVITY

That 'a man is an old as his arteries' was stated first by Thomas Sydenham, a 17th-century physician. That 'a man's arteries are as old as he makes them' was stated by Robert Bell, a 19th-century physician. Perhaps we can proceed one step further to state the obvious: the arteries and all the organs and tissues are as young as the cells of which they are made and the *milieu interieur* which sustains them.

Diet is not the only factor in longevity, of course, but it is by far the main one. The closer we can get to an ideal diet and maintain it, the less will be the wear and tear on our organs and the slower the accumulation of the fibrinous, gelatinous growths and calcareous mineral salts in our cells and tissues.

Think of all those little cells. Dr Edward J Stiegbitz, MS MD FACP, in his book *The Second Forty Years*, says:

... superficially, the answer is simple; intrinsically, extremely complex. Whether the cells themselves are, or are not, potentially immortal is largely beside the point. The essential fact is that continuance of such perpetual youth, as displayed by Carrel's chick heart cultures, is absolutely dependent upon the maintenance of an ideal environment. Cultures must be aseptically transplanted to fresh media at frequent intervals or growth stops and the cells die, poisoned by the accumulating chemical debris of their living, and starved because their foodstuffs are used up. Contamination with even minute amounts of toxic substances or any inadequacy of any one of many nutritional requisites immediately interrupts the marvellous lifestream. The quality of the cellular environment is the determining factor, whether the cells be growing in vitro in a test-tube, or in vivo, in the living and functioning organism.*

Do the best you can

Your body is a living and functioning organism and you want it to stay that way. You know what to do. We have discussed at great length the factors responsible for polluting the *milieu interieur* of the body and to eliminate

* Steigbitz's reference chick heart cultures was in relation to the experiments begun in 1912 by Dr Alexis Carrel, at the Rockefeller Institute in New York, in which Carrel kept alive some cells taken from the heart tissue of an embryo chicken. Properly nourished and cleansed, the cell culture thrived and appeared to be immortal, at least until 1947 when the experiment was terminated.

them would appear to be easier said than done. Not everybody can arrange to live in a tropical Garden of Eden.

We can only do our best with what we have available, and the first step, wherever your live, is to cut down on the things that do the most harm. Eat as much as you can of your food raw. Cut out salt. Think of those little cells. Think of how clean your arteries will be, how comforting it will be never to worry about cancer. Each step you take will improve your wellbeing and increase your life expectancy.

Think of fruit as sustaining food and not just an accessory adding colour to the sideboard. The quality of the fruit is important: much of the commercially grown fruit available today looks a lot better than it tastes, and lack of taste means lack of nutrition and possibly at the same time the presence of insecticide traces.

Do the best you can, remembering Dr De Lacy Evans' words of wisdom:

There is, therefore, a simplicity, a reason, a wonderful philosophy in the first command given to man — man may live entirely upon fruits in better health than the majority of mankind now enjoy. Good, sound, ripe fruits are never the cause of disease, but the vegetable acids, as we have before stated, lower the temperature of the body, decrease the process of combustion or oxidation — therefore the waste of the system — less sleep is required, activity is increased, fatigue or thirst is hardly experienced; still the body is well nourished, and as a comparatively small quantity of earth salts are taken into the system, the cause of old age is in some degree removed, the effect is delayed, and life is prolonged to a period far beyond our 'threescore and ten'.

CHAPTER 11

In conclusion

'The problem of cancer must be considered as an insoluble medical problem, because it is essentially a nutritional and social problem, in other words a problem of prevention. Such a problem cannot be solved by animal experiments, vaccines and drugs. Statisticians, pathologists, biochemists and doctors cannot solve social problems.'
— Kasper Blond, English cancer specialist

There is no mystery about cancer. Cancer is a natural physiological process that follows strict biological laws: it is none other than a predictable response of normal body cells to a disordered state of the bloodstream in which situation they are forced to revert to a more primitive form in order to survive individually.

The biological laws are understood. The factors leading to the disordered situation are understood. The sequence of events is understood. The factors that worsen the situation and the factors capable of improving the situation are understood and are controllable.

These points conceded, it is obvious that cancer is easily preventable and, if corrective action is taken in its early stages, is easily reversible.

Remember, the greatest influence on the purity or impurity of your blood — on your general health and span of life — is the sort of food you eat. A sound constitution, supported by correct dietary habits, ensures a healthy bloodstream and healthy tissues.

Cancer cannot occur in healthy tissues.

Cigarette smoke may damage your lungs, so might asbestos particles; sunlight may damage your skin and so might a variety of chemicals — but cancer will not ensue, not in healthy tissue.

The body has enormous reserves and powers of recuperation — assets which diminish with age. Proper eating habits will preserve these assets and prolong your life. What other benefits can you expect? Plenty. If reasonable care is taken, allowing for occasional wayward excursions, you will not only be cancerproof, you will find you no longer get colds in summer or winter, you will have no aches and pains, no asthma, and no arthritis any more. You will be free from heart disease, eye problems, PMT, prostate disorders, and so on. Blow your doctor a kiss.

You will have achieved homeostasis and with it rejuvenation. You will have more money to spare and more time in which to spend it. Bon voyage.

Appendixes

APPENDIX A

THE PRIME CAUSE AND PREVENTION OF CANCER

BY OTTO WARBURG, DIRECTOR OF THE MAX PLANK INSTITUTE
FOR CELL PHYSIOLOGY, BERLIN-DAHLEM, GERMANY
Lecture at the meeting of the Nobel-Laureates on 30 June 1966
at Lindau, Lake Constance, Germany. English edition by Dean Burk,
National Cancer Institute, Bethesda, Maryland

Cancer, above all other diseases, has countless secondary causes. But, even for cancer, there is only one prime cause. Summarised in a few words, the prime cause of cancer is the replacement of the respiration of oxygen in normal body cells by a fermentation of sugar. All normal body cells meet their energy needs by respiration of oxygen, whereas cancer cells meet their energy needs in great part by fermentation. All normal body cells are thus obligate aerobes, whereas all cancer cells are partial anaerobes. From the standpoint of the physics and chemistry of life this difference between normal and cancer cells is so great that one can scarcely picture a greater difference. Oxygen gas, the donor of energy in plants and animals is dethroned in the cancer cells and replaced by an energy yielding reaction of the lowest living forms, namely, a fermentation of glucose.

The key to the cancer problem is accordingly the energetics of life, which has been the field of work of the Dahlem institute since its initiation by the Rockefeller Foundation about 1930. In Dahlem the oxygen transferring and hydrogen transferring enzymes were discovered and chemically isolated. In Dahlem the fermentation of cancer cells was discovered decades ago; but only in recent years has it been demonstrated that cancer cells can actually *grow in the body almost with only the energy of fermentation.* Only today can one submit, with respect to cancer, all the experiments demanded by Pasteur and Koch as proof of the prime cause of a disease. If it is true that the replacement of oxygen respiration by fermentation is the prime cause of

159

cancer, then *all* cancer cells without exception must ferment, and no normal growing cell ought to exist that ferments in the body.

An especially simple and convincing experiment performed by the Americans Malmgren and Flanegan confirms this view. If one injects tetanus spores, which can germinate only at very low oxygen pressures, into the blood of healthy mice, the mice do not sicken with tetanus, because the spores find no place in the normal body where the oxygen pressure is sufficiently low. Likewise, pregnant mice do not sicken when injected with the tetanus spores, because *also in the growing embryo no region exists* where the oxygen pressure is sufficiently low to permit spore germination. However, if one injects tetanus spores into the blood of tumour-bearing mice, the mice sicken with tetanus, because the oxygen pressure in the tumours can be so low that the spores can germinate. These experiments demonstrate in a unique way the anaerobiosis of cancer cells and the *non-anaerobiosis of normal cells*, in *particular the non-anaerobiosis of growing embryos*.

The fermentation of Morris hepatomas

A second type of experimentation demonstrates a quantitative connection between fermentation of tumours and growth rate of tumours.

If one injects rats with cancer-inducing substances of different activities, one can create, as Harold Morris of the National Cancer Institute in Bethesda has found, liver cancers (hepatomas) of very different degrees of malignancy. Thus, one strain of tumour may double its mass in three days, another strain may require 30 days. Recently Dean Burk and Mark Woods, also of the National Cancer Institute, measured the *in vitro* rates of anaerobic fermentation in different lines of these hepatomas, and obtained a curve (Figure 1) that shows a quantitative relationship between fermentation and growth rate, and therefore between fermentation and malignancy, in these various tumour strains. The fermentation increases with the malignancy, and indeed the fermentation increases even faster than the malignancy.

Special interest attaches to the fermentation of the most slowly growing hepatomas, because several investigators in the United States believed that they had found[1] that such tumours had no fermentation, which would have meant that there exist tumours growing without fermentation; that is, that anaerobiosis cannot be the prime cause of cancer.

Dean Burk and Mark Woods saw immediately from their curves that in the region of the zero point the rate of fermentation was so small that it could no longer be measured by the usual gross methodology employed by the aforementioned workers, whereas in the same region the smallest growth rate was always easily measurable. Burk and Woods saw, in other words, that in the region of the zero point of their curves the growth test

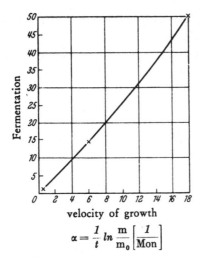

$$\alpha = \frac{1}{t} \, ln \, \frac{m}{m_0} \left[\frac{1}{Mon}\right]$$

Figure 1: Velocity of growth and fermentation of the Morris hepatomas, according to Dean Burk and Mark Woods

was more sensitive that the *usual* fermentation test. With refined and adequate methods for measuring fermentation of sugar (glucose) they found, what any physical chemist after a glance at the curve would realise, that even the most slow-growing Morris hepatomas fermented sugar.

The results of Dean Burk and Mark Woods were confirmed and extended by other workers with independent methods. Pietro Gullino also in Bethesda, developed a perfusion method whereby a Morris hepatoma *growing in the living animal* could be perfused for long periods of time, even weeks, by means of a single artery and single vein, and the blood entering and leaving any given tumour could be analysed. Gullino found with this method that the slow-growing Morris hepatomas always produced fermentation lactic acid during their growth. This was in contrast to liver, where, as known since the days of Claude Bernard, lactic acid is not produced but consumed by liver; the difference between liver and Morris tumours *in vivo* is thus infinite (+ vs. –). Gullino further found that tumours grow *in vivo* with diminished oxygen consumption. In summary, Gullino's findings indicate that the slow-growing Morris hepatomas, are partial anaerobes. Silvio Fiala, a biochemist at the University of Southern California, found that not only did the slow-growing hepatomas produce lactic acid, but also that the number of their oxygen-respiring grana was reduced.

The slow-growing Morris hepatomas are therefore far removed from having refuted the anaerobiosis of tumours. On the contrary, they are the best proof of this distinctive characteristic. For forty years cancer investigators have searched for a cancer that did not ferment. When finally a non-fermenting tumour appeared to have been found in the slow-growing Morris tumours, it was shown to be a methodological error.

Transformation of embryonic metabolism into cancer metabolism

A third type of experiment, from the institute of Dahlem with coworkers Gawehn, Geissler and Lorenz, is likewise highly pertinent. Having established that anaerobiosis is that property of cancer cells that distinguishes them from all normal body cells, we attached the question, how normal body cells may become transformed into anaerobes.

If one puts embryonic mouse cells into a suitable culture medium saturated with physiological oxygen pressures, they will grow outside the mouse body, *in vitro*, and indeed as pure aerobes, with a pure oxygen respiration, without a trace of fermentation.

However, if during the growth one provides an oxygen pressure so reduced that the oxygen respiration is partially inhibited, the purely aerobic metabolism of the mouse embryonic cells is quantitatively altered within 48 hours, in the course of *two* cell divisions, into the metabolism characteristic of fermenting cancer cells. Figure 2 illustrates the very simple experimental procedure involved.

If one then brings such cells, in which during their growth under reduced oxygen pressure a cancer cell metabolism has been produced, back under the original high oxygen pressure, and allows the cells to grow further, the cancer metabolism *remains*. The transformation of embryonic cell metabolism into cancer cell metabolism can thus be irreversible, an important result, since the origin of cancer cells from normal body cells is an irreversible process. It is equally important that these body cells whose metabolism has thus been transformed into cancer metabolism now continue to grow *in vitro* as facultative anaerobes. The duration of our experiments is still too limited to have yielded results of tests of inoculation of such cells back into mice, but according to all previous indications such cells will later grow as anaerobes upon transplantation into animals.

In any case, these experiments belong to the most important experiments in the field of cancer investigation since the discovery of the fermentation of tumours. For cancer metabolism, heretofore measured so many thousands of times, *has now been induced artificially in body cells* by the simplest conceivable experimental procedure, and with this artificially induced cancer metabolism the body cells divide and grow as anaerobes *in vitro*.[2]

In recent months we have further developed our experimental arrangements so that we can measure manometrically the oxygen respiration and fermentation of the growing mouse embryonic cells

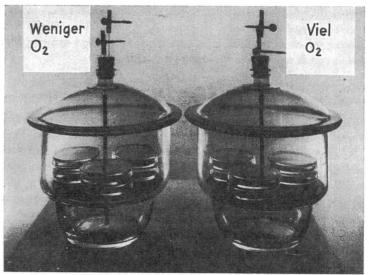

Figure 2: Method to transform embryonic metabolism into cancer metabolism by decreasing the oxygen pressure

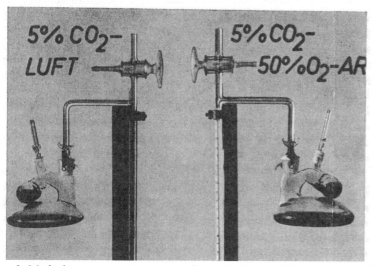

Figure 3: Method to measure manometrically respiration and fermentation during the transformation of embryonic into cancer metabolism[4]

during the metabolic transformation. Figure 3 shows the experimental arrangement. We find by such experiments that 35% inhibition of oxygen respiration already suffices to bring about such a transformation during cell growth.[3] Oxygen pressures that inhibit respiration 35% can occur at the end of blood capillaries in living animals, so that the possibility arises that cancer may result when too low oxygen pressures occur during cell growth in animal bodies.

The induction of cancers by solid materials injected into animals is a further experimental indication of this possibility. If one implants discs of solid substances under the skin of rats, the discs will soon be surrounded by capsules of living tissue that will be nourished with blood vessels from the hypodermis. Sarcomas very frequently develop in these capsules. It is immaterial whether the solid discs are chemically plastics, gold or ivory, etc. What produces the cancer is not the chemical nature of the solid discs, but the special kind of blood nourishment supplied to the tissue encapsulating the discs. This blood provision varies with the site and inadequacy within a given animal, and induces cancer from the low oxygen pressure in the encapsulating disc.

Thermodynamics
If a lowered oxygen pressure during cell growth may cause cancer, or, more generally, if any inhibition of respiration during growth may cause cancer, then a next problem is to show *why* reduced respiration induces cancer. Since we already know that with a lowering of respiration fermentation results, we can re-express our question: Why does cancer result if oxygen-respiration is replaced be fermentation?

The early history of life on our planet indicates that life existed on earth before the earth's atmosphere contained free oxygen gas. The living cells must therefore have been fermenting cells then, and, as fossils show, they were undifferentiated single cells. Only when free oxygen appeared in the atmosphere — some billion years ago — did the higher development of life set in, to produce the plant and animal kingdoms from the fermenting, undifferentiated single cells. What the philosophers of life have called 'Evolution créatrice' has been and is therefore the work of oxygen.

The reverse process, the de-differentiation of life, takes place today in greatest amount before our eyes in cancer development, which is another expression for de-differentiation. To be sure, cancer development takes place even in the presence of free oxygen gas in the atmosphere, but this oxygen may not penetrate in sufficient quantity into the growing body cells, or the respiratory apo-enzymes of the growing body cells may not be saturated with the active groups. In any case, during the cancer development the oxygen-respiration always falls, fermentation appears, and the highly differentiated cells are transformed to fermenting anaerobes, which have lost all their body functions and retain only the now useless property of growth. Thus, when respiration disappears, life does *not* disappear, but the *meaning* of life disappears, and what remains are growing machines that destroy the body in which they grow.

But why oxygen differentiates and why lack of oxygen de-differentiates? Nobody would dispute that the development of plants and animals and man from unicellular anaerobes is the most improbable process of all processes in the world. Thus there is no doubt, that Einstein descended from a unicellular fermenting organism — to illustrate the miracle, molecular O_2 achieved. But according to the thermodynamics of Boltzmann, improbable processes require work to take place. It requires work to produce temperature differences in a uniformly temperatured gas; whereas the equalisation of such temperature differences is a spontaneous process that does not require work. It is the oxygen-respiration that provides in life this work, and de-differentiation begins at once when respiration is inhibited in any way. In the language of thermodynamics, differentiation represents a forced steady state, whereas de-differentiation — that is, cancer — is the true equilibrium state. Or, illustrated by a picture: the differentiated body cell is like a ball on an inclined plane, which would roll down except for the work of oxygen-respiration always preventing this. If oxygen respiration is inhibited, the ball rolls down the plane to the level of de-differentiation.

But why respiratory energy and not fermentation energy can differentiate, whereas in general, for example in growth, respiratory energy and fermentation energy are equivalent? *Obviously, there would be no cancer* if there were not this discrimination of fermentation energy, that is, *if fermentation like respiration could differentiate*. Then, when respiration is replaced by fermentation, fermentation would take over differentiation, and a high state of differentiation would be maintained even in the fermenting body cells.

Chemistry
Physics cannot explain why the two kinds of energy are not equivalent in differentiation; but chemistry may explain it. Biochemists know that both respiration energy and fermentation energy do their work as phosphate energy, but the ways of phosphorylation are different. If one applies this knowledge to carcinogenesis, it seems that only oxidative phosphorylation but not fermentative phosphorylation can differentiate, a result, that may in future explain the mechanism of differentiation.

Yet Biochemistry can explain already today why fermentation arises, when respiration decreases. Figure 4 shows that the pathways of respiration and fermentation are common as far as pyruvic acid. Then the pathways diverge. The end product of fermentation is reached by one single reaction, the reduction of pyruvic acid by dihydro-nicotinamide to lactic acid. On the other hand, the end products of the oxidation of pyruvic acid, H2O and CO2, are only reached after many additional reactions.

Therefore, when cells are harmed, it is probable that first respiration is harmed.

$$\text{Glucose} + 4H_3PO_4 = 2 \text{ diphosospho-glycerialdehyde}$$
$$\text{Diphosospho-glycerialdehyde} + \text{nicotinamide} =$$
$$\text{Diphosospho-glyceric-acid} + \text{Dihydro-nicotinamide} =$$
$$\text{Pyruvic acid} + \text{dihydro-nicotinamide}$$

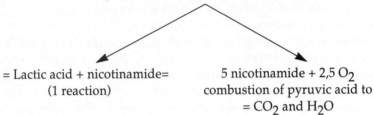

= Lactic acid + nicotinamide=	5 nicotinamide + 2,5 O_2
(1 reaction)	combustion of pyruvic acid to
	= CO_2 and H_2O

Figure 4

To sum up:

1. Impairment of respiration is more frequent than impairment of fermentation because respiration is more complicated than fermentation.
2. The impaired respiration can be easily replaced by fermentation, because both processes have a common catalyst, the nicotinamide.
3. The consequence of the replacement of respiration by fermentation is mostly glycolysis, with death of the cells by lack of energy. Only if the energy of fermentation is equivalent to the lost energy of respiration, is the consequence anaerobiosis. Glycolysis means death by fermentation, anaerobiosis means life by fermentation.
4. Cancer arises, because respiration, but not fermentation, can maintain and create the high differentiation of body cells.

To conclude the discussion on the prime cause of cancer, the virus-theory of cancer may be mentioned. It is the most cherished topic of the philosophers of cancer. If it were true, it would be possible to prevent and cure cancer by the methods of virology; and all carcinogens could be eaten or smoked freely without any danger, if only contact with the cancer virus would be avoided.

It is true that some virus-caused cancers[5] occur in animals, but not one sure human virus-cancer has been observed so far, whereas innumerable substances cause cancer without viruses in animals and man. Thus viruses do not meet the demands of Pasteur, that it must be possible to trace the prime cause in every case of the disease. Therefore science classifies viruses as remote causes of cancer, leading to anaerobiosis, the prime cause, that meets the demands of Pasteur.

Many may remember how anaerobiosis as prime cause of cancer was recently disputed emphatically, when one single cancer — the slow Morris hepatomas — was believed (wrongly) to lack in fermentation. In contrast the virus theory is adhered to although all cancers of man are lacking in virus-origin. This means the surrender of the principles of Pasteur and the relapse into bygone times of medicine.

Applications

Of what use is it to know the prime cause of cancer? Here is an example. In Scandinavian countries there occurs a cancer of the throat and oesophagus whose precursor is the so-called Plummer-Vinson syndrome. This syndrome can be healed when one adds to the diet the active groups of respiratory enzymes, for example: iron salts, riboflavin, nicotinamide, and pantothenic acid. When one can heal the precursor of a cancer, one can prevent this cancer. According to Ernest Wynder of the Sloan-Kettering Institute for Cancer Research in New York, the time has come when one can exterminate this kind of cancer with the help of the active groups of the respiratory enzymes.

It is of interest in this connection that with the help of *one* of these active groups of the respiratory enzymes, namely nicotinamide, tuberculosis can be healed quite as well as with streptomycin, but without the side effects of the latter.[6] Since the sulphonamides and antibiotics, this discovery made in 1945 in the most important event in the field of chemotherapy generally, and encourages, in association with the experiences in Scandinavia, efforts to prevent cancer by dietary addition of large amounts of the active groups of the respiratory enzymes. Since there can scarcely be overdosage, such experiments can do no harm.

I would like to go further and propose always making dietary additions of large amounts of the active groups of the respiratory enzymes after successful operations when there is danger from metastatic growths. One could indeed never succeed in re-differentiating the de-differentiated cancer cells, since during the short duration of human life the probability of such a back-differentiation is zero. But one might increase the respiration of growing metastases, and thereby inhibit their fermentation, and — on the basis of the curve of Dean Burk and Mark Woods obtained with the Morris hepatomas — thereby inhibit the growth of metastases to such an extent that they might become as harmless as the so-called 'sleeping' cancer cells in the prostates of elderly men.

A second example of application

The physicist Manfred von Ardenne has recently attacked the problem of the therapy of cancer. Ardenne discovered that cancer cells owing to their fermentation, are more acid — inside and on their surface — than normal cells and hence are more sensitive to high temperatures. On this basis, he and his medical colleagues have treated cancer patients, after surgical removal of the primary tumours, by raising the body temperatures of the patients to about 109° Fahrenheit for an hour, in the hope that the metastases will then be killed or their growth so slowed up as to become harmless. It is not yet decided whether this idea can be described as a practical success. But the provisional work of Ardenne is already of great significance in a field where hopes of conventional chemotherapy have been dimmed but might be brightened by combination with extreme or moderate hyperthermy.

A third application. According to an estimate by K H Bauer of the Cancer Institute in Heidelberg, at least one million of the now living twenty five million male inhabitants of West Germany will die of cancer of the respiratory tract; still more will die from other cancers. When one considers that cancer is a permanent menace, one realises that cancer has become one of the most dangerous menaces in the history of medicine.

Many experts agree that one could prevent about 80% of all cancers in man, if one could keep away the known carcinogens from the normal body cells. This prevention of cancer might involve no expenses, and especially would require little further research to bring about cancer prevention in up to 80%.[7]

Why then does it happen that in spite of all this so little is done towards the prevention of cancer? The answer has always been that one does not know what cancer or the prime cause of cancer be, and that one cannot prevent something that is not known.

But nobody today can say that one does not know what cancer and its prime cause be. On the contrary, there is no disease whose prime cause is better known, so that today ignorance is no longer an excuse that one cannot do more about prevention. That prevention of cancer will come there is no doubt, for man wishes to survive. But how long prevention will be avoided depends on how long the prophets of agnosticism will succeed in inhibiting the application of scientific knowledge in the cancer field. In the meantime, millions of men must die of cancer unnecessarily.

Notes

1. For example see C H Bohringer Son, Ingelheim am Rhein, the factory work journal Das Medizinische Prisma, vol. 13, 1963. Here a lecture of Van Potter (Madison, Wisconsin) is reprinted where owing to the slow-growing Morris-tumours anaerobiosis as prime cause of cancer is rejected and the lack of 'intracellular feedback' is claimed to be the real cause of cancer.

2. These experiments were at once repeated, when they were published …
   without acknowledgment …
3. These experiments show, like the curve of Dean Burk and Mark Woods in
   Figure 1 [velocity of growth and fermentation of Morris hepatomas], that
   it is more correct to designate tumour cells as 'partial anaerobes' rather
   than 'facultative anaerobes'. A body cell is transformed into a tumour cell
   if only a part of the respiration is replaced by fermentation.
4. The vessels are not shaken, because shaking inhibits growth. Therefore
   the oxygen pressure in the liquid phase at the bottom of the vessels is
   much lower than in the gasphase. For example, when the oxygen pressure
   in the gasphase was 2000 mm H_2O it was at the bottom of the vessels
   130 mm H_2O. (O Warburg, A Geissler and S Lorenz, Zeitschr, für
   Naturforschung 20 b, 1070, 1965.)
5. The chicken Rous sarcoma, which is labelled today as a virus tumour,
   ferments glucose and lives as a partial anaerobe like all tumours.
6. V Chlorine: C R sci Paris, 220, 150 (1945). H Fust und A Studer,
   Schweizerische Z für allgemeine Pathologie, Band 14; Fasc 5 (1951).
7. Since this estimate was published, some thought 80% even too low. Yet
   prevention remained taboo and early diagnosis was the only consolation
   that was offered.

Source: Otto Warburg, 'The prime cause and prevention of cancer, with two prefaces on prevention', revised lecture of the meeting of the Nobel Laureates on 30 June 1966 at Lindau, Lake Constance, Germany' (2nd revd edn), English edition by Dean Burk), published by Konrad Triltsch, Würzburg, Germany, 1969.

APPENDIX B

THE MEDICAL TREATMENT OF CANCER

'Considered in its broadest terms, orthodox cancer treatment today is a failure and a disgrace. Contemporary cancer management in a number of respects, constitutes professional malpractice.'
— Dr Brian A Richards, *The Topic of Cancer*, 1982

'Surgery brings a mechanical approach to a biological problem.'
— Dr Miles Little, Professor of Surgery, University of Sydney

'Our failure to improve survival rates has been due to clinicians rigidly maintaining obsolete concepts of the nature of the disease.'
— Dr M Baum, *British Medical Journal*, 1976

'There is no evidence that mastectomy affects survival. If women knew that they would probably refuse surgery.'
— Dr L Cunningham, *Lancet*, 1980

'The evidence that breast cancer is incurable [that is, by medical means] is overwhelming. The philosophy of breast cancer screening is based on wishful thinking that early cancer is curable cancer, though no one knows what is "early" ... Adherence to these myths and avoidance of reality undermines the credibility of the medical profession with the public ... If breast cancer is incurable, as many surgeons believe, then screening only adds years to anxiety and fear ... It is unacceptable to remove breasts on the basis of theoretical speculation.'
— Dr P Skrabanek, *Lancet*, 1985

'The difference between incidence and mortality suggests that no improvement in survival has occurred as a result of surgery.'
— D J Benjamin, CSIRO scientist, 1993

'When we look back at what we do to cancer today, chopping it out, burning it out, poisoning it out, it will all seem so crude.'
— Dr Robert Good, Former Director of the
Sloan Kettering Institute

'Success of most chemotherapies is appalling ... There is no scientific evidence for its ability to extend in any appreciable way the lives of patients suffering from the most common organic cancer ... chemotherapy for malignancies too advanced for surgery which accounts for 80% of all cancers is a scientific wasteland.'
— Dr Ulrich Abel, Hippocrates Verlag, Stuttgart, 1990

'If I contracted cancer, I would never go to a standard treatment centre. Cancer victims who live far from such centres have a chance.'
— Professor George Mathe, French cancer specialist,
Medicines Nouvelles, March 1989

In the last ten years, since the 4th edition of *The Health Revolution* was published, the only significant change in the field of cancer is the death rate: it has increased from one in five to one in four in the Western world, and continues to increase. How could it be otherwise as our dietary transgressions continue to worsen, while politicians think health problems can be solved by more taxes, and while doctors, grateful for their status and income, put on a brave front that (given the resources) medical science will soon solve all problems?

EXCERPT FROM THE HEALTH REVOLUTION
In a lecture at the American Cancer Society's annual Science Writers' Conference in New Orleans in 1969, Dr Hardin Jones of the University of California Department of Medical Physics, said:

> My studies have proven conclusively that untreated cancer victims actually live up to four times longer than treated individuals. For a typical type of cancer, people who refused treatment lived for an average of twelve and a half years. Those who accepted surgery and other kinds of treatment lived an average of only three years ...

In a paper titled 'Cancer cures more deadly than disease', Dr Jones said further:

It is utter nonsense to claim that catching symptoms early enough will increase the patient's chances of survival. Not one medical scientist or study has proven that so in any way. Furthermore, untreated breast cancer cases show a life expectancy four times longer than treated ones. My wife and I have discussed what she would do if breast cancer were diagnosed in her, and we both agree she would do nothing except to keep as healthy as possible. I guarantee she would live longer. For not only does radical surgery or chemotherapy do nothing to prolong a cancer victim's life, but that same person will, in most cases, live a lot longer if he or she refuses treatment. Beyond a shadow of doubt, radical surgery on cancer patients does more harm than good.

The continued failure to effectively combat cancer, despite the repeated optimistic promises of new breakthroughs has reduced the credibility of the medical profession, but this failure is made to look less dismal by the misleading survival rates published by medical authorities. Because a patient who remains free of symptoms for five years is considered to be 'cured' of cancer, medical statistics of cure rate do not reflect the true situation. When relatively harmless skin cancers are included as well, the overall cure rate for cancer appears much better still. It is obvious that the earlier cancer is detected in the first place the more chance a patient has of meeting the five-year criterion, but in fact this does not extend the patient's life, it merely makes the statistics look better.

Conventional medical treatment of cancer is a failure for the obvious reason that it is not addressed at removing the cause but merely at destroying one of the symptoms, i.e. the cancer growth. This absurdity is due to the steadfastly held view that cancer occurs as a local malfunction of cell growth caused probably by a chance mutation in an otherwise healthy body. The other symptoms of weight loss, fatigue, poor skin tone, etc. are thought to be caused by the tumour growth.

The three basic medical treatments are surgery, radiation and chemotherapy, all of which are traumatic and more often than not accelerate the decline of the patient.

Whereas there may be something gained by the surgical removal of a self-contained tumour inasmuch as stopping its parasitic action, in most cases there are millions of stray cancer cells already circulating in the body and usually metastases already established. When a surgeon says 'he got it all' he is being very optimistic.

Dr Robert Bell, MD FRPS, formerly a cancer surgeon who abandoned surgery when he realised its futility against cancer and devoted the rest of his life to natural healing, wrote: 'It is of no more avail to excise the local manifestation of blood contamination — which cancer undoubtedly is —

and thus expect to eradicate the constitutional affliction, than it is to cut out a piece of dry rot in a beam without adopting means to remove the cause of the mischief.'

Furthermore, surgery or biopsy, because the subsequent healing process causes de-differentiation of tissue cells, can actually initiate cancer growth. In such cases, said Sir James Paget, 'The surgeon has unwittingly supplied by the local injury what was needed for the production of a cancerous growth.'

After surgery, radiation and/or chemotherapy is the next step, because even in 'terminal' cases, it is hoped that by retarding the tumour growth, the patient will gain extra time. Radiation usually diminishes the size of the tumour, and this is encouraging to see, but once again this is only the diminution of a symptom. While this is going on, destruction occurs to normal tissue as well, and enormous numbers of circulating white cells of the immune system are destroyed.

Said Dr W A Dewey, Professor of Therapeutics, University of Michigan: 'As radium is directed only at the end products of cancer, it is not only useless, but it destroys the healthy tissue around the tumour, destroying blood vessels and protective glands which are most necessary to the healing process, and chases the disease to some internal organ, thus so complicating the case that cure is impossible.'

Chemotherapy is even worse. US Senator Humphrey before he died, called it 'death in a bottle'. The idea of chemotherapy is to delay cancer growth by preventing replication of the cells, and the so-called 'advantage' of the chemicals is that they circulate through the entire body so reaching all sites of cancer growth whether detected or not. The disadvantages are that all other replicating normal cells are affected as well, resulting in hair loss and ulceration of various tissues, accompanied by nausea, vomiting, vertigo and so on. At the same time, the already diminished immune system is further destroyed.

It is hard to believe. The medical authorities and the chemical manufacturers admit that the chemicals used can actually cause cancer, and the pharmacists who handle them wear special protective clothing and masks in fear of their own lives. These frightening chemicals are then purposefully injected into the very bloodstream of the cancer patient, whose wretched liver now has to try to detoxify this further assault. As the patient's survival depends upon restoration of the liver and the functioning of the immune system, chemotherapy is not only bound to fail, it virtually guarantees the patient's further decline.

On chemotherapy, Dr Charles Huggins, Nobel Prize winner, of the University of Chicago, said: 'I am very much against chemotherapy generally. It simply makes the patients too ill. Remember there are worse things than death. One of them is chemotherapy.'

Sometimes radiation and chemotherapy are used together, and this procedure is the most lethal of all, but is commonly used by doctors obsessed with the destruction of cancer cells regardless of all else. Hope rises as the tumour diminishes in size, and then crashes as the inevitable regrowth appears.

The entire medical show, nothing less than ridiculous when honestly assessed, is of course fearfully expensive in money, and in terms of grief and despair, immeasurable.

At the Annual Scientific Meeting on the Subject of Cancer at Sydney University in November 1980, Dr P Shubik of America was frank. In his opening remarks he said: 'there were no cancer experts any more in the USA'. What he meant was that cancer has the medical profession perplexed and confused (in 1995 they are still perplexed and confused). There is no medical cure presently foreseen, and hope lies mostly in extending the life of patients by improving current methods of treatment. During the meeting, the subjects of diet, physical fitness, exercise and stress were not discussed except for one 'workshop' on diet to which only two doctors attended. During the meeting (which I attended), the immune system was discussed once, but not as a serious cancer factor.

More recent are reports of the work of Professor John Williams' team at the Australian National University in Canberra. Hoping for a breakthrough, they are seeking methods of arresting cachexia, the wasting of the body which occurs in the final stages of cancer. A medical breakthrough will only be achieved however when the fact, known for over a hundred years, is accepted that not only cachexia, but the tumour, the pre-cancer and the 'cancer milieu' are all stages of the one degenerative process.

Why are people still ignorant of medical facts known for one hundred years or more?

In addition to Drs Koch, Gerson and Moerman, there have been a whole successions of doctors going right back to Dr Lambe in 1908 who have successfully treated cancer by helping their patients correct the constitutional disorders of their bodies.

Despite their proven methods, these doctors could never break the barrier of prejudice historically surrounding the medical profession, but instead were persecuted in varying degrees as troublesome non-conformists. Such rejection is a peculiar part of human nature and has always been encountered by innovators in all fields.

For a new method to be accepted by the medical establishment, the fact that it works is almost irrelevant. Unless research is on an 'in' subject and conducted on 'approved' lines, the authors of research papers have great difficulty having them printed, particularly in the more conservative medical journals. Dr Gerson submitted dozens of papers on cancer therapy to the Journal of AMA but none were accepted. Dr Koch and Dr Moerman, along with Dr Hoxsey and many others, received the same rejection.

This is why today the medical profession is so ignorant of much vital information, not only information on cancer. The vital facts of diabetes and heart disease also, known for over one hundred years and scientifically proven in the 1930s by Dr I M Rabinowitch and in the 1940s by Dr Lester Morrison, are still unknown to most doctors.

This opposition and cover-up is due not only to conservatism and vested professional interests, it is professed policy of the drug and chemical corporations together with such food industries as the meat, dairy and sugar industries who between them control most of the funding for medical research.

Hopefully the orthodox medical establishment will eventually get the message. In her book *Cancer Under Siege*, Dr June Goodfield quoted Dr Robert Good, director of the Sloan-Kettering Institute as saying: 'When we look back at what we do to cancer today, chopping it out, burning it out, poisoning it out, it will all seem so crude.'

Dr Good, why do you think Dr de Lacey Evans and Dr Bell gave up surgery a hundred years ago?

Let Dr Kasper Blond sum it up. He said: 'The problem of cancer must be considered as an insoluble medical problem, because it is essentially a nutritional and social problem; in other words a problem of prevention. Such a problem cannot be solved by animal experiments, vaccines and drugs. Statisticians, pathologists, biochemists and doctors *cannot solve social problems.'*

Source: Ross Horne, *The Health Revolution* (4th edition), Happy Landings, Sydney, 1985, pages 277–81.

CANCER UPDATE 1995

From 26 to 30 June 1995 the *Sydney Morning Herald* ran a series of articles on cancer, based on interviews with a number of leading cancer researchers and physicians. These articles, by the *Herald*'s medical writer, Melissa Sweet, contained some disturbingly bad news together with some encouraging good news:

> Cancer is now the major cause of premature death in Australia, killing one person every 17 minutes.
>
> New research by the NSW Cancer Council reveals that in 1991 cancer accounted for 42% of deaths in Australian females aged under 70, and 31% of premature male deaths. The findings, to be published in July's [1995] *Cancer Forum* journal, show that in the same year cancer caused more than

50 per cent of all deaths in women aged between 40 and 60, and a total of 31,609 Australian deaths.

Associate Professor Richard Taylor, head of the NSW Central Cancer Registry and one of the report's authors, said it was the first to show that cancer has overtaken cardiovascular disease to become the major cause of premature death in this country.

Now the good news:

> The authors of the report say: 'Cancer is Australia's most important health problems. Many of the people who are dying of this disease are productive members of society with young families. There is an urgent need to reassess priorities for prevention and control in order to address these facts.'

The good news doesn't sound much, but the final sentence provides the enouragement: 'There is an urgent need to reassess priorities for prevention and control ...' The operative word is *reassess*, an admission that previously held ideas have been wrong and that a sensible evaluation of long-neglected information is now possible.

Commenting on the situation, Martin Tattersall, Professor of Cancer Medicine, Sydney University, said that many treatments have not been properly evaluated or are ineffective, largely because research and treatment agendas are often set by the pharmaceutical industry rather than in the patients' best interests. He said doctors' vested interests also often determine the type of treatment that patients receive. The *Herald* article went on to say:

> Despite the explosion of scientific knowledge about cancers due to modern techniques of molecular biology, some doctors say it is unrealistic to expect an overall cure will ever be found. Many note that `Magic Bullet' treatments and immunotherapy have failed to live up to expectations, and also doubt whether the widely heralded gene therapies will deliver their promise.
>
> The process which makes cells start growing out of control is still not fully understood and nor is the interaction between environmental factors such as diet and the genetic changes involved in cancer. Doctors, for the most part, are not able to predict which patients will relapse or which cancers will become resistant to treatment.
>
> 'For most people, we can't say why they develop the cancer,' says Professor Michael Friedlander, Director of the Institute of Oncology, Prince of Wales Hospital.
>
> Professor Miles Little, a Professor of Surgery at the University of Sydney, says the public has a media-driven perception that medicine is a deterministic science that can provide black and white answers. 'The nature of medical knowledge in relation to cancer is actually very weak. What we rely on to a great extent is a series of observations,' he says. `We observe that

a certain percentage will survive, but we can't determine who those people will be. Practically all of cancer is based on this.'

Professor Stephen Leeder, a Professor of Community Medicine and Public Health at the University of Sydney, argues that the medical profession and society need to take a whole new appproach to cancer. First, he says, there needs to be frank acknowledgment that the news about cancer is grim and that the efforts to date 'have been picking away at the margins'. He says the NSW Cancer Council campaign to promote positive messages with the slogan 'cancer is a word, not a sentence' is 'very silly' and ignores the reality of cancer.

He also says many doctors wrongly 'skate over' depressing survival figures for fear it will alarm people and claims that specialists, despite genuine concerns for patient welfare, also have a vested interest in maintaining the popularity of attempted curative treatments. 'I don't think that any of us like statistics being advanced which suggest that what we are doing isn't working,' he says.

Leeder says we need to develop a new concept about cancer. Instead of putting so much effort into attempting to cure, we should learn to live with it and focus more on improving patients' quality of life.

Right-oh, are we agreed it's back to the drawing board?

Dr Bell, Dr Gerson, Dr Koch, Dr Warburg, Dr Burk and Dr Moerman were men born ahead of their time. They put the data on the drawing board a long while ago but *now their time has arrived.*

APPENDIX C

THE DUBIOUS VALUE OF MAMMOGRAMS AND HORMONE REPLACEMENT THERAPY

MAMMOGRAMS

Currently in Australia medical authorities are conducting an intensive campaign urging all women over the age of 50 years to have regular mammograms to detect if they have breast cancer in an early stage as yet not large enough to be felt as a lump.

The object of this campaign is commendable because it is intended to save lives, in the belief that the earlier cancer can be detected, the greater the possibility of a cure. This belief is valid and absolute commonsense, but *only if correct procedures are followed*.

Conventional medical procedures are to be deplored, and are counter-productive to the potentially valuable early warning provided by a positive mammogram. The only correct procedure therefore (whether a mammogram result is positive *or* negative) is to avoid attacking a suspected symptom and to concentrate on correcting the cause.

The following information was provided by the journal of the US National Health Federation, *Health Federation News* (January 1995).

In November 1992, the Canadian National Breast Screening Study, the most comprehensive such study to date, was published. It involved following for seven years almost 90,000 women; 50,000 were aged 40–49 years, and about 40,000 were aged 50–59 years. Half of both groups received yearly ordinary breast exams plus mammograms. The other half received only ordinary breast exams — a single breast exam if they were 40–49, or an annual breast exam if they were 50–59.

In the seven years of follow-up of the two groups of younger women, 38 women who had the annual mammogram plus physical exam died of breast cancer, compared with 28 deaths in the group that had only a single physical exam at the beginning.

In the seven years of follow-up of the two groups of older women, there was no difference in the death rates.

So the conclusion of the study, containing in all just on 90,000 women, was that mammography provided no advantage over a yearly physical breast exam.

This is not to say that mammography is not effective. It is. It can detect cancer too small to be felt by touch, but the interpretation of the results is not always clear-cut, and false positives do occur, all of which lead to further medical procedures that as likely as not do more harm than good.

In the National Health Federation article 'Do mammograms save women's lives?', Dr Julian Whitaker MD, of California, said:

> Women are more frightened of breast cancer than any other disease, and for many, yearly mammograms have become routine. Promoters of this screening test assure women that frequent mammograms save lives. It is an easy sell.
>
> I used to routinely recommend mammography to my patients over 50, but not any more. I now think a routine mammogram is a waste of time and money, and instead of saving lives will only stimulate a lot of unnecessary surgery that leaves physical and psychological scars. Even more serious, the resources gobbled up by the proliferation of mammography centres will continue to delay serious study and education on how to prevent breast cancer.
>
> This is bad, especially as there is so much women can do on their own to protect themselves from breast cancer. Preventive techniques such as diet modifications, avoidance of pesticides and other industrial waste products, and the use of antioxidant vitamins and minerals, particularly Vitamin A and selenium, and perhaps just eating a raw sprig of broccoli each day, in my opinion, would save far more lives than the annual mammogram given to millions of women in this country.
>
> Just like all disease-screening programs, mammography generates a lot of activity. Women who receive mammograms have roughly twice as much cancer diagnosed, twice as many surgical procedures, open biopsies, needle biopsies, many more benign biopsies, and a slight increase in the use of mastectomy. With all this activity we should be seeing some reduction in the death rate from breast cancer. But we are not.

Pointing out that medicine is an industry run on commercial lines, Dr Whitaker said further:

> Every industry this size is a predictable spokesman for itself and is likely to counter any negative information. As you would expect, the American College of Radiology, the physicians most intimately involved in this industry, openly advocate mammography for all women over 40. However, the government funded National Cancer Institute (NCI) is back-pedalling on its recommendations. Advisory committees are pressuring the NCI to recommend mammography screening only for women over 50, every one or two years. But the American Cancer Society [ACS] is holding firm on its recommendation for young women to have a yearly mammogram beginning

at age 35, simply ignoring the Canadian study that is clearly the most informative study yet published.

Personally, I think a lot of the folks down at the ACS should hit the pavement and look for some honest work.

I am particularly concerned that the cancer 'establishment' and even our own President, label mammograms and other screening techniques as 'preventive medicine'. These techniques are early detection methods and are no more effective at preventing cancer than watering your lawn is at preventing automobile accidents.

It's understandable that the President could confuse detection with prevention, but not the cancer establishment. I believe they deliberately misuse the language to cover their backsides for not paying attention to preventive techniques.

As for early detection, I do not plan to recommend mammography to my female patients with negative breast exam, although I will educate them on the issues and let them make their own decision. I do urge an annual breast exam and to perform a self-exam each month. If you are still menstruating, do these self-exams two or three days after your period ends, if you are no longer menstruating, pick a day each month that will serve as a reminder. Combined with disciplined use of preventive techniques this is the best defence against breast cancer.

(Dr Whitaker of California was among the first doctors to recognise the immense importance of the achievements of Nathan Pritikin in reversing coronary artery disease in hundreds of patients at the Longevity Centre in Santa Monica at the time in 1975 when the American medical establishment was labelling Pritikin as a quack. Dr Whitaker is also the author of the books *Reversing Health Risks* and *The Heart Surgery Trap*.)

HORMONE REPLACEMENT THERAPY
The relationship between production of hormones and intake of fat
The human body, when in good health, is as robust and durable as that of any other member of the animal world. Unfortunately, however, due to the various bad habits — mainly dietary bad habits — that civilised humans have managed to invent, the people who indulge in these bad habits sooner or later show the evidence of wear and tear in the form of various health problems.

The worst of the many harmful substances contained in our traditional Western diet is fat, and whereas most nutritionists agree that ideally fat in the diet should not exceed 10% of the total energy value (kilojoules) in the diet, the typical modern diet contains about 40%. It is this intake of fat which is the prime cause of most of the 'diseases of civilisation', the major ones being heart disease and other circulatory problems, cancer, arthritis, asthma, migraine, pre-menstrual tension, diabetes, prostate and menopausal problems. Regardless of what doctors believe about heredity and the unavoidability of these problems, it is a simple matter to arrest and in most cases reverse these ailments simply by strict dietary correction. And very quickly too, as I have explained at length in my several books.

Oestrogen and progesterone are the female sex hormones, and their production in the body is influenced by the level of fat in the diet. It is the highly excessive level of fat in the modern diet compared with the simpler diets of many years ago that causes the abnormal production of these hormones and premature sexual development of females, and their larger bosoms, that occurs today. Whereas in years past girls began to menstruate at age about sixteen, today they begin at about twelve.

It is the excess fat that is also responsible for the almost universal weight problems of today with the accompanying increased risk of every disease in the book, including cancer, particularly breast cancer, which is strongly influenced by hormone levels.

Hormone replacement therapy, osteoporosis and breast cancer
Another problem more prevalent among women today is osteoporosis, the weakening of bones by their loss of calcium, supposedly caused by the lowered production of oestrogen that occurs after menopause. The real reason for osteoporosis is that the body withdraws calcium from the bones in an effort to neutralise the acidic nature of the blood consequential to excess levels of dietary protein and salt. The condition is made worse by lack of exercise, by smoking and by various medical drugs such as thyroid hormones and corticosteroid tablets.

Tests described by Dr Kenneth Cooper, the man who evolved the Aerobic exercise program, showed that in a six-month test, women supplied with supplementary calcium actually lost more calcium from their bones, whereas those on an exercise program only, with no supplementary calcium, in fact gained bone density.

Dietary correction, of course, is the real answer — vegetarians as a rule, do not experience osteoporosis. Researchers at the University of Texas Health Science Centre have observed that a diet rich in animal protein increases calcium loss by nearly 50% compared to a vegetarian diet, and other researchers at the University of California have noted in tests on rats that a diet high in fat and sugar also results in loss of bone density. Dr Singer of the National Osteoporosis Foundation, on the subject of salt, stated: 'If you take an animal and put him on a high salt diet, he will lose bone. No question.'

In a large-scale study of eating habits in China, Dr Colin Campbell, of

Cornell University, found that bone density problems occur only in those parts of China where people consume foods high in animal protein — including milk. In areas where people were mainly vegetarian there was little or no osteoporosis.

Along with osteoporosis it is also the now common lack of oestrogen after menopause that is held responsible for the other distressing symptoms that occur — such as hot flushes, night sweats, mental problems, sleeplessness, bladder problems and the increased danger of blood clots and heart attacks — and it has been shown that hormone replacement therapy (HRT) may help to relieve some of these symptoms. For this reason the therapy is becoming widely used.

However, many medical research doctors are extremely suspicious of HRT because there are too many inconsistencies and conflicting data about it as well as evidence that shows HRT results in a significantly increased risk of cancer. And whereas HRT supposedly protects against osteoporosis, has been pointed out that hip fractures from osteoporosis is just as common among men as it is in women, having increased threefold in the last thirty years. Moreover it is a fact that *the lowest incidence of heart disease occurs in countries where women's oestrogen levels are the lowest, as it is also with cancer.*

In Britain most of the women who submit to HRT discontinue it, according to Guy's Hospital in London, the reasons being bleeding, feeling bloated, weight gain, nausea, breast tenderness and headaches, as well as concern about cancer and effects as yet unknown.

Other 'therapies'

What follows is hard to believe, but true — it has been proposed by some medical scientists that, in order to prevent breast cancer, pre-menopausal women be routinely treated with a drug, GnRH, which affects the pituitary gland so to prevent the production of oestrogen and progesterone. And then, because this results in menopausal effects in young women, they are given a certain amount of artificial oestrogen replacement therapy to prevent these effects, and a course of synthetic progesterone every fourth month to ensure their continued fertility, which means they only have menstrual periods three times a year! On a trial of this 'preventive therapy', women on the GnRH treatment experienced severe osteoporosis, losing 2% of their bone mass in less that a year!

A ten-year trial by the US Federal Government National Cancer Institute, involving 16,000 supposedly healthy women over age 35, has been in progress since early 1992. This trial, called the Breast Cancer Prevention Trial, is designed to determine whether the drug tamoxifen effectively prevents the disease. A sum of US$70 million has been allocated to this trial on the flimsy evidence that, out of eight previous studies, only one study suggested any benefit could accrue to pre-menopausal women who took the drug, while at the same time another study showed that cancer risk was actually increased by the drug. To make things worse, it is already known that tamoxifen causes a sevenfold increase in the incidence of blood clots, and increases the risk of endometrial cancer as much as five times, but the director of the trial says that this risk is no greater than it would be on oestrogen therapy, but he did not add that endometrial cancer caused by tamoxifen was much deadlier, causing liver damage as well.

By now you are probably slowly shaking your head in wonderment at the absurd behaviour of supposedly intelligent people and you no doubt would shake all over if you knew of the complicity between various 'custodians of public health' and the pharmaceutical companies whose marketing methods make the cigarette companies look like amateurs and whose legal drugs cause more harm than all the illegal ones put together.

The alternative to HRT
The alternative to HRT is to get healthy and fit and then throw all your medicines into the sea, whereupon — as Doctor Oliver Wendel Holmes once said — 'it would be so much better for man, and so much the worse for the fishes'.

APPENDIX D

EXCERPT FROM THE *GERSON HEALING NEWSLETTER*

FROM CHARLOTTE GERSON'S CLINICAL NOTEBOOK
Endometriosis

We are so blessed with uncounted numbers of recovered cancer patients that we are often specially happy to share with our members dramatic patient stories who have recovered from other diseases.

This week, two such patients came to our attention: Judy S, back in 1986, was suffering terrible pain from endometriosis. In January 1986, she submitted to a laparoscopy only to have a definite diagnosis of her problems. She was suffering from very severe pain, especially during her ovulation, on urinating and moving her bowels. Her menstruations, too, were usually abnormal, passing large clots, too short bleeding or too long. One day after her laparoscopy, she started on the Gerson Therapy. She refused all 'orthodox' treatments. After about one month, she started to have less pain; she says the coffee enemas helped. Soon, her menstrual periods became more normal, and she stopped bleeding at ovulation time. Before the therapy, this bleeding at ovulation sometimes lasted 10 days. The endometrium had overgrown and was attached to the ovaries and the back of the uterus. After six months on the Gerson Therapy, she had no more pain at all and her periods were normal.

On the first try, she became pregnant — but due to unwise counsel she stopped the Therapy and added salt and fat to her diet. She had three normal pregnancies and nursed all her babies 16–17 months.

Now she has some recurrence of her endometriosis — but since she knows what to do, the enemas help her overcome pain, and she went back on the complete, less intensive Therapy. She says that this time, she will stay on it for 1½ years to get well and stay well.

The unusual twist to this story is that Judy tells me that her mother-in-law, Frances S, was a patient of Dr Gerson's for a benign cyst. Her son (Judy's brother-in-law), Todd, had muscular dystrophy and was treated by Dr Gerson. He is now, at 40, cured and completely normal.

At a very recent Health Convention we attended in Chicago, we met a lady (Anna K) who came all the way from Detroit to be with us. She told her story which sounds almost incredible — but I know that all kinds of miracles are possible on the Gerson Therapy. Also, when I study her problems a little more closely, many of them relate to a damaged immune system. This could easily be partly due to her fluoridated water in Detroit. I incredulously listened to her story.

She was so ill, weak and non-functional that, when she heard of the Gerson Therapy and heard that I would be giving a lecture and seminar in Miami, she travelled all the way from Detroit to attend. She was convinced and impressed and embarked on the Gerson Therapy for herself in September 1991 to overcome these problems: endometriosis, allergies, sinus infections, chronic bronchitis, chronic kidney infections (she stated that she thought these were hereditary since her mother suffered from the same problem), inner ear ulcers, chronic fatigue — with loss of memory and concentration, ocular migraines (these affect vision, causing blurring, etc.), arthritis, heart valve problems, stomach ulcers, fungus (candida).

She reports that she is doing extremely well and feels strong and healthy, says she is no longer suffering from any of the above symptoms, has good energy and concentration. Frankly, she really looks well and fit.

That is not the end of the story!

She tells that she also has a son — Yogi, now 18 — who, she says, had the following problems: ear infections from birth and was treated with antibiotics, allergies, severe constipation (moved bowels once a week), migraines, intermittent high fevers, strep infections.

He also did the Gerson Therapy, which is difficult for teenagers because of peer pressure. But he is so well now, he has become an instructor in self-defence, and urges his students to change their diet for better energy, concentration and control.

ANTIHISTAMINES

One of our supportive physicians, familiar with Gerson Therapy, recently made the following remark: 'It is interesting and rather alarming that most of the intricacies of the human metabolic biochemistry is poorly understood. Also, most of the actions of drugs and effect on this complex biochemistry, are poorly understood. Yet, orthodox medicine uses these drugs with the greatest abandon — regularly causing new problems and dislocations in the body biochemistry.'

This statement is well illustrated by an item we found recently in the Scientific News page of the *International Herald Tribune* [19 May 1994]:

US TESTING THREE ALLERGY DRUGS
Washington (AP) — Tests by Canadian researchers showing that three common allergy drugs promote cancers in laboratory mice has prompted the

US Food and Drug Administration to begin its own investigation of the prescription antihistamines. Neither the researchers nor the FDA advised consumers to stop taking the drugs although they cautioned against long term use. The FDA noted that no clinical studies to determine the effect on humans had yet been conducted and that only certain antihistamines were implicated in the Canadian study. The principal Canadian researcher, Dr Lorne J Brandes, said that so far, benefits of antihistamines appear to outweigh the risks.

In the study published in the Journal of the US National Cancer Institute, Dr Brandes and his research team at the Manitoba Institute of Cell Biology in Winnipeg injected mice with a skin cancer and a cancer of the connective tissue, known respectively as melanoma and fibrosarcoma. In three different groups of mice, the tumours grew faster and larger after the rodents were injected with one of three antihistamines; loratadine, astemizole and hydroxyzine, all of which are prescription drugs.

When we looked up 'histamines' and 'antihistamines' in the classic medical text *Pathology*, by Stanley L Robbins, MD, we find the following statement: 'Histamine is present in many tissues. Its job in normal cells is not fully understood.' Further down, we read: '... most cells, too, release histamine, though for what purpose in normal life we do not know.' Then, the author goes on to state: 'Antihistamine drugs in small doses inhibit the specific effects of histamine and delay, but do not prevent the development of the inflammatory exudate.'

Dr Gerson regularly describes the importance, especially in cancer patients, of inflammation, and described that inflammation fluid (exudate) helps to kill cancer cells! So, it seems quite logical that antihistamines tend to aggravate cancer — or worse. Yet, the medical authorities feel that the benefits of these drugs outweigh its possible dangers.

The other item found on the same page of the *International Herald Tribune* (19 May 1994) is also an indictment of the usual medical advice to patients to obtain an early diagnosis. It implies quite clearly that one might do best to leave certain cancers alone rather than to mutilate the patient!

PROSTATE SURGERY EFFECTS
Dallas (AP) — Men who have their prostate gland removed because of early signs of cancer run a higher than expected risk of losing urinary control and the ability to have sex, the study concludes.

The study, conducted at Harvard affiliated hospitals, found that the side effects of this common operation are much more frequent than surgeons usually acknowledge. The report is the latest contribution to the controversy over how — and even whether — prostate cancer should be diagnosed and treated. An estimated 200,000 cases, 80% of them at early stages, will be diagnosed this year in the United States.

The study was directed by Dr James Talcott of Dana-Farber Cancer Centre in Boston. He presented his findings at a meeting of the American Society of Clinical Oncology.

USE THE RIGHT JUICER

Dr Gerson's urging to use the right juicer: confirmed once again!

At the beginning of May, we received a phone call from Colleen C of Syracuse, NY. She was told that she was only the 4th person in medical history to be diagnosed with a melanoma in the nose. She continued: 'They wanted to take my teeth, gums, bone under the eye and above the eye, cut my face open and radiate my face — but not put anything back — very deforming, face sunken!' She didn't want any part of that.

She found out through a friend about the Gerson Therapy, got the Gerson book and realised 'This was it!'

She started the Therapy with a centrifugal juicer for seven weeks and found that her tumour remained steady but there were no significant changes. On 'Good Friday', she started the Therapy with the proper juicer. After 4 weeks, she 'blew a tumour out of her nose'. Her skin colour went from orange to whitish, energy level increased. She was amazed at the dramatic changes with the right juicer. Her friends are organising a fund raiser for her so she can go to the Hospital.

Only about a week later, during my one day's stay in London, a lady showed up at my lecture there. She told virtually the same story; She had uterine cancer and started the therapy with a centrifugal juicer — nothing happened for about 8 months! A short while after getting a loan of a Champion juicer, and making her juice with it, she had a strong healing reaction and is now well on her way to a total recovery.

CAN WE GET ENOUGH PROTEIN ON A TOTALLY VEGETARIAN DIET?
Patient story by Howard Straus, Editor

We are often asked whether we are getting enough protein on a totally vegetarian diet. Americans have been generally convinced by the purveyors of meat and dairy products that they need animal protein to have enough energy for athletic performance.

In fact, most vegetables are very high in protein, with the notable exception of yams and sweet potatoes. As far as athletic performance and stamina are concerned, our performance fuel is complex carbohydrates. The following story is illustrative.

At a recent POWER NUTRITION seminar, Dianna S, now recovered over five years on the Gerson Therapy from recurrent breast cancer, told us of one experience she had while she was on the therapy.

After a year and a half of therapy, with little exercise other than juicing, Dianna, then 53, felt well enough to go down to her tennis club to see if she could scare up a match. She loves tennis and had played very well before her illness.

At the club there was a women's singles tournament beginning, and when she was invited to join, she did so with a little trepidation, as she had not conditioned herself.

She won her first match, a hard fought, three set match. She paused for lunch, which she had brought with her. She then proceeded to win her afternoon match more easily.

Having won, Dianna was now required to play in the semifinals the following day! In the past she would have been wiped out for days after an intense match, but, to her great surprise, she felt terrific. Not only did she win the semifinal match, but before the final, she played three hard sets of mixed doubles. In the end, she won the club championship and felt no fatigue or exhaustion the next day. And this after over eighteen months of the virtual inactivity required by the Therapy. Her stamina and energy remain higher than that of her 28 year old daughter. You may not become a tennis champion like Dianna, but we can assure you that you are more than adequately provided with protein!

VITAMIN RICH FOODS BEHIND CANCER RECOVERY — STUDY
Paul Clayton and Judy Jones
Reprinted from the *Edmonton Journal*, Thursday, 28 April 1994:

Women with breast cancer may significantly improve their chances of recovery by changing their diet, new research suggests.

A group of Danish sufferers has experienced marked improvements in health since they began taking dietary supplements rich in vitamins and minerals, in addition to routine treatments.

All 32 women had advanced tumours when they embarked on the trial in Copenhagen two years ago. Six would have been expected to die during that time under normal circumstances. Instead, all have survived and sustained modest or dramatic improvement in their conditions.

The specialists who ran the trial have hailed the results as an important breakthrough in the treatment of breast cancer.

The critical role of diets rich in fruit and raw or lightly cooked vegetables in helping to prevent cancer and heart disease has been accepted by growing numbers of doctors and scientists.

The Danish research provides a strong indication that diet can also help to control and even eradicate cancer, as well as prevent it.

None of the women in the breast cancer trial lost weight during the two years, and they needed fewer pain killers than would be expected. None of them experienced any spread of the cancer. Three of the women were cured and a further three experienced a substantial regression of their tumour. Most said they had felt much better since embarking on the trial.

In addition to receiving radiotherapy, chemotherapy or surgery — or a combination of these — the women were put on an intensive program of dietary supplements. These consisted of the anti-oxidants vitamins C, E and betacarotene; selenium, a trace mineral; fatty acids such as those commonly found in fish oils, and a branded formulation of a substance known as Vitamin Q, which the body makes naturally from other vitamins. Previous studies have shown that levels of Vitamin Q in cancer patients are abnormally low.

The selection of dietary supplements was made after an analysis of all the available scientific literature on the anti-cancer effects of all vitamins and minerals.

'I have never before seen a spontaneous regression of the type of breast tumours that we were treating in this trial,' said cancer specialist Dr Knud Lockwood.

PANCREATIC CANCER WITH LIVER METASTASES
Patient letter, from Kay

Dear Charlotte

I thought I would write you this letter to let you know how Ron is doing as well as to thank you for the inspiration you gave us when we were down at CHIPSA eight months ago.

We know you talk to hundreds of cancer patients every week and it must be almost impossible to remember them all. To refresh your memory: we were down at CHIPSA in June, 1993. Ron was diagnosed with pancreatic cancer with metastases to the liver. He was 45 years old and had taken no other conventional treatments before coming to CHIPSA. After we had been doing the therapy at home for 6 weeks, you came up to Seattle for the NHF convention, and Ron spoke to the audience during your presentation, testifying to how well he felt with the therapy.

Anyway, Ron is currently at 8½ months on the therapy and doing very well. He has gained all his weight back, has no abdominal pain, has high energy and looks terrific! We recently had an ultrasound done on him and the mass that was clearly visible in the head of the pancreas last year is no longer visible now! The lesions in the liver are larger this year, but are surrounded by dark rims which we are hoping is inflammatory fluid and a sign that the body is now working on those tumours. (Comment: more likely they represent encapsulation — Charlotte.) His doctor is pleased and needless to say, so are we.

This therapy has certainly turned our world upside down. Our lives are necessarily structured totally around Ron's therapy and survival. I've become quite creative as a vegetarian cook and we have curious onlookers from our community all the time. Ron and I were invited to speak at a local community college (where I took my nursing school) and he captivated the audience and enlightened them as well.

Thank you again for carrying on the vital work of your father and for offering hope to all those cancer patients that were given no hope before. We plan to see you in Seattle again this year if you're up here again!

Ron & Kay

'Study Nature, its eternal laws will keep you'
— Dr Max Gerson to his daughter.

Source: *The Gerson Healing Newsletter*, July–August 1994. (The newsletter is the membership organ of the Gerson Institute. For details, write to: The Gerson Institute, PO Box 430 Bonita, California USA 91908–0430.)

APPENDIX E

THE HISTORY OF THE PEDESTAL TOILET

The toilet first became popular in England in approximately 1850, and its use soon spread throughout the civilised world. It caught on quickly because it came on the scene at the same time as plumbing, which allowed for clean disposal of what had previously been stored in chamber pots or dumped in the street.

The toilet was originally designed by Joseph Bramah, a cabinet maker, and improved upon by Thomas Crapper, a plumber. These were not men of medicine, and did not recognise the mechanical advantage that squatting offers the body. Nor was the general public aware, which is why the toilet became the norm before we knew it.

It was not until the early 1900s that wise doctors, faced with dramatically increased incidence of disease, questioned the conventions of the time — and the convention most suspect was the toilet. In one book written in 1924, called *The Culture of the Abdomen*, the author quoted leading medical authorities of the time who were very outspoken about the toilet's faulty design and ensuing health consequences. He states, 'It would have been better if the contraption had killed its inventor before he launched it under humanity's buttocks.

Constipation, hernias, varicose veins, haemorrhoids and appendicitis were all attributed to the use of the toilet. A solution to the dilemma was offered in the form of a footstool used to elevate the feet to the approximate squatting posture. At one point, the footstool was so popular it was being sold at Harrod's of London. [Similar footstools are available by mail order in Australia and the USA.]

Source: William Welles, DC, 'The importance of squatting', *Natural Health Society Journal*, Penrith NSW.

Select bibliography

INTRODUCTION
Australian Broadcasting Corporation (ABC). *Understanding Cancer*, television program, 1984.

CHAPTER 1: THE HUNZAS
Hilton, James. *Lost Horizon*, Macmillan, London, 1933.
McCarrison, Sir Robert. Cited by G T Wrench, in *The Wheel of Health*, C W Daniel & Co, London, 1938.

CHAPTER 2: HEALTHY BLOOD, HEALTHY CELLS, HEALTHY BODY
Banik, Allen E. *Hunza Land*, Whitehorn Publishing Co, Long Beach, California, 1960.
Cannon, Walter. *The Wisdom of the Body*, W W Norton, 1932.
Knisely, Melvin H. 'Sludged blood' and 'Intravascular erythrocyte aggregation: blood sludge', in *Handbook of Physiology: Circulation III*, 1963.

CHAPTER 3: WHAT IS CANCER?
Bell, Robert. *The Cancer Scourge and How to Destroy It*.
Israel, Lucien. *Conquering Cancer*, Random House, New York, 1978.
Moerman, Cornelius. *A Solution to the Cancer Problem*, C Moerman, Vlaardingen, Netherlands, 1962; English translation published by The International Association of Cancer Victims and Friends Inc., Los Angeles, 1962.
Owens, Guy. Cited in Raymond K Brown, *AIDS, Cancer and the Medical Establishment*, Robert Speller Publisher, New York, 1986.

CHAPTER 4: WHO GETS CANCER AND WHO DOESN'T?
Bernstein, Leslie. Breast cancer study at the University of California, reported in *Journal of the National Cancer Institute*, vol. 86, 1994, pages 1403–8.
Dungal, Neils. 'Stomach cancer in Iceland', a lecture presented at the meeting of the International Academy of Pathology, Chicago, 26 April 1961, and later reported in *Journal of the American Medical Association*.
Frisch, R E. Study of the prevalence of breast cancer, reported in *British Cancer Journal*, 1985.
Gerson, Max. *A Cancer Therapy: Results of Fifty Cases*, Totality Books, Delmar, California, 1958; distributed by the Gerson Institute, Bonita, California.
Horne, Ross. *Improving on Pritikin*, Happy Landings, Avalon Beach NSW, 1988.

Multiple Risk Factor Intervention Trial (US), evaluated in the *Journal of the American Medical Association*, January 1987.

National Research Council (US), *Diet, Nutrition and Cancer*, National Academy Press, Washington DC, 1982.

Natural Food and Farming, Atlanta, Texas.

Nossal, G J. *Antibodies and Immunity*, Nelson, 1968.

Ogilvie, Heneage. *No Miracles Among Friends*, Parrish, London, 1959.

Scharffenberg, J A. Article on smoking in *Life and Health*, 1979.

Stamler, Jeremiah. Lecture on a study conducted by Loma Linda University, California, on Seventh Day Adventists, published in *Circulation*, July 1978.

Tipper, E H. *The Cradle of the World and Cancer*, 1927.

CHAPTER 5: SOME CANCER THEORIES

Australian Broadcasting Corporation (ABC), *Understanding Cancer*, television program, 1984.

Garten, Max. *Civilised Diseases and their Circumvention*, Macmillan World Publishers, San Jose, California, 1978.

Horne, Ross. *Health and Survival in the 21st Century*, Margaret Gee Publishing, Sydney, 1992.

Horne, Ross. *The Health Revolution* (4th edn), Happy Landings, Avalon Beach NSW, 1985.

Israel, Lucien. *Conquering Cancer*, Random House, New York, 1978.

Issels, Joseph. *Cancer: A Second Opinion*, Hodder & Stoughton, London,1975.

Pauling, Linus, & Cameron, Ewan. *Cancer and Vitamin C: A Discussion of the Nature, Causes, Prevention and Treatment of Cancer with Special Reference to the Value of Vitamin C*, Warner Books, New York, 1979.

Walser, Mackenzie. Cited in Ross Horne, *The Health Revolution* (4th edn), Happy Landings, Avalon Beach NSW, 1985.

CHAPTER 6: EXPLAINING CANCER

Bell, Robert. *Cancer, Its Cause and Treatment Without Operation*,1903.

Bell, Robert. *The Cancer Problem in a Nutshell, Cancer and its Remedy*, Methuen, London, 1912.

Bell, Robert. *The Cancer Scourge and How to Destroy It*, Health Seekers International, Pinetown, South Africa.

Bell, Robert. *Health at its Best Versus Cancer*.

Bell, Robert. *The Reminiscences of an Old Physician*, Murray, London, 1924.

Burk, Dean. `New approaches to cancer therapy', *New England Natural Food Bulletin*, Spring, 1974.

Burk, Dean, & Woods, Mark. Cited in Otto Warburg, 'The prime cause and prevention of cancer, with two prefaces on prevention', revised lecture of the meeting of the Nobel Laureates on 30 June 1966 at Lindau, Lake

Constance, Germany' (2nd revd edn), English edition by Dean Burk, published by Konrad Triltsch, Würzburg, Germany, 1969. (Provided as Appendix A.)

Dintenfas, Leopold. *Blood Micro-rheology Viscosity Factors in Blood Flow, Ischemia and Thrombosis*, Butterworth Press, 1971.

Dintenfas, Leopold. *Blood Viscosity in Heart Disease and Cancer*, Pergamon Press, 1981.

Dintenfas, Leopold. *Rheology of Blood in Diagnostic and Preventative Medicine*, Butterworth Press, 1976.

Garten, Max. *Civilized Diseases and Their Circumvention*, Macmillan World Publishers, San Jose, California, 1978.

Gerson, Max. *A Cancer Therapy: Results of Fifty Cases*, Totality Books, Delmar, California, 1958; distributed by the Gerson Institute, Bonita, California.

Goldblatt, H, & Cameron, G. *Journal of Experimental Medicine*, vol. 97, 525, 1953.

Hassan, Mulhim. *Prevention and Cure of Cancer*, Exposition Press, New York, 1983.

Issels, Joseph. *Cancer: A Second Opinion*, Hodder & Stoughton, London, 1975.

Knisely, Melvin. *Life* magazine, 31 May 1948.

Koch, William F. *The Survival Factor in Neoplastic and Viral Diseases*, Vanderkloot Press, Detroit, 1961.

Life magazine, 31 May 1948.

Michaels, L. Cited in Leopold Dintenfas, *Rheology of Blood in Diagnostic and Preventative Medicine*, Butterworth Press, 1976.

Moerman, Cornelius. *A Solution to the Cancer Problem*, C Moerman, Vlaardingen, Netherlands, 1962; English translation published by The International Association of Cancer Victims and Friends Inc., Los Angeles, 1962.

Stinkvist , Bjorn. Cited in Ross Horne, *The Health Revolution* (4th edn), Happy Landings, Avalon Beach NSW, 1985.

Warburg, Otto. 'The prime cause and prevention of cancer, with two prefaces on prevention', revised lecture of the meeting of the Nobel Laureates on 30 June 1966 at Lindau, Lake Constance, Germany' (2nd revd edn), English edition by Dean Burk, published by Konrad Triltsch, Würzburg, Germany, 1969. (Provided as Appendix A.)

Windesch, F. *Experimental Medicine*, vol. 97, no. 525, 1953.

Wood, Summer. *AMA Archives of Pathology*, vol. 66, October 1958.

CHAPTER 7: MORE ON DIET AND OTHER FACTORS

Ahlson, Charles B. *Health from the Sea and Soil*, Exposition Press, New York, 1962.

Aldercreutz, Hermann. *Health Freedom News* (Journal of the US National Health Federation), January 1995.

American Dental Association News, 31 July 1972.

Aviles, Professor. 'The anti-cancerous properties of vitamin F', *Let's Live*, September 1954.

Bagnall, Victor. 'Nutrition: its relation to cancer', cited in Ross Horne, *The Health Revolution* (4th edn), Happy Landings, Avalon Beach NSW, 1985.

Barnes, Broda. *Hypothyroidism: The Unsuspected Illness*, Harper & Row, New York, 1976.

Berg, John. Cited in Ross Horne, *The Health Revolution* (4th edn), Happy Landings, Avalon Beach NSW, 1985.

Black, H S, et al. *New England Journal of Medicine*, vol. 330, no. 18, May 1994, pages 1272–5, cited in *Vantage Point*, vol. 4, no. 8, 1994.

Blond, Kasper. *The Liver and Cancer: A New Cancer Therapy*, 1955.

Brandes, Lorne. Cited in the *Gerson Healing Newsletter*, July-August 1994.

British Cancer Institute. Cited in Ross Horne, *The Health Revolution* (4th edn), Happy Landings, Avalon Beach NSW, 1985.

British Ministry of Health. Cited in Wendy Varney, *Fluoride in Australia: A Case to Answer*, Hale & Iremonger, Sydney, 1986.

Brody, Jane, & Holleb, Arthur. *You Can Fight Cancer and Win*, McGraw Hill, New York, 1977.

Burkitt, Denis, & Trowell, Hugh. Lectures at the Pritikin Research Institute, Santa Barbara, 1976.

Carroll, Kenneth K. 'Experimental evidence of dietary factors and hormone-dependent cancers', *Cancer Research*, vol. 35, page 3379.

Coulter, Harris. *AIDS & Syphilis: The Hidden Link*, North Atlantic Books, Berkeley, California, 1987.

Dean Burk Foundation. Open communication, 10 December 1983.

Evans, Charles De Lacy. *How to Prolong Life: An Enquiry into the Cause of Old Age and Natural Death* (1879), Charles Sawyer, London, 1910.

Fluoride Question: Panacea or Poison? Stein & Day, New York, 1975.

Gerson, Max. *A Cancer Therapy: Results of Fifty Cases*, Totality Books, Delmar, California, 1958; distributed by the Gerson Institute, Bonita, California.

Gibbons, De Lamar. Cited in *Gerson Healing Newsletter*, May–June 1994.

Goth, A, & Littmann, I. 'Ascorbic acid content in human cancer tissue', *Cancer Research*, vol. 8, 1948.

Hall, M G. 'Faecal bile acids and clostridea in patients with cancer of the large bowel', *Lancet*, 8 March 1975.

Hall, M G. 'Steroid nuclear dehydration and colon cancer', *American Journal of Clinical Nutrition*, 27 December 1974.

Health Freedom News (Journal of the US National Health Federation), January 1994. Report on osteoporosis and fluoride.

Heinerman, John. Cited in *Gerson Healing Newsletter*, May–June 1994.

Heinerman, John. *The Treatment of Cancer with Herbs*, Biworld Publishers, Orem, Utah, 1980.

Hetzel, B. Cited in Ross Horne, *The Health Revolution* (4th edn), Happy Landings, Avalon Beach NSW, 1985.

Horne, Ross. *Health and Survival in the 21st Century*, Margaret Gee Publishing, Sydney, 1992; Chapter 7, 'AIDS, yuppie flu and the common cold'.

Howell, Edward. *The Status of Food Enzymes in Digestion and Metabolism*, National Enzyme Co, Chicago, 1946.

Hoxsey, Harry S. *You Don't Have to Die*, Milestone Books, New York, 1956.

Issels, Joseph. *Cancer: A Second Opinion*, Hodder & Stoughton, London, 1975.

Journal of the American Medical Association, 18 September 1943. Report on the distribution of fluorine.

Journal of the National Cancer Institute, October 1993. Report on the link between prostate cancer and the eating of meat and fat.

Kalokerinos, Archie, & Dettman, Glen. *Second Thoughts About Disease*, Biological Research Institute, Warburton, Vic., 1977.

Kenney, Joy. *Pritikin Vantage Point*, vol.4, no.7, July 1994.

Kouchakoff, Paul. 'The influence of food cooking on the blood formula of man', paper delivered to First International Congress of Microbiology, Paris, 1930.

Kunin, Richard. *Meganutrition*.

Lane, William Arbuthnot. *The Prevention of the Diseases Peculiar to Civilisation*, 1929.

Livingstone, Virginia. *Cancer: A New Breakthrough*, 1972.

McKenna, Joan. Correspondence with Professor Peter Duesberg UCB, 1990.

Mainlow, M R. Cited in Ross Horne, *The Health Revolution* (4th edn), Happy Landings, Avalon Beach NSW, 1985.

Mendelsohn, Robert. *The Confessions of a Medical Heretic*, Contemporary Books, Chicago, 1979.

Moskowitz, Richard. 'Immunisations: a dissenting view', in Robert S Mendelsohn, George Crile, Samuel Epstein, Henry Heimlich, Alan Scott Levin, Edward R Pinckney, David Spodick, Richard Moskowitz & George White, *Dissent in Medicine: Nine Doctors Speak Out*, Contemporary Books, Chicago, 1985.

Multiple Risk Factor Intervention Trial (US), evaluated in the *Journal of the American Medical Association*, January 1987.

Murray, Maynard. *Sea Energy Agriculture*, Valentine Books, Winston-Salem, North Carolina, 1976.

Nathan Pritikin Lecture, 1984.

National Cancer Institute. *Journal of National Cancer Institute*, October 1993.

Nature, December 1978. Report on animal experiment showing that dietary cholesterol paralyses the macrophages.

Netherlands Cancer Institute study by Dr Flora E van Leeuwen.

Netherlands Cancer Institute, research on the pill and breast cancer, reported in *Lancet*.

New England Journal of Medicine, vol. 330, 1994. Figure illustrating the incidence of actinic keratosis. Report on vitamin A therapy in male smokers in Finland.

New England Journal of Medicine, May 1994. Report by the Meyer L Pentis Comprehensive Cancer Centre, Michigan, on dietary fat as the major factor in prostate cancer.

Ogilvie, Heneage. *No Miracles Among Friends*, Parrish, London, 1959.

Okomura, T, & Matsuhisha, T. Cited in George L Waldbott, *Fluoridation: The Great Dilemma*, Coronado Press, Lawrence, Kansas, 1978.

Paget, Sir James. Quoted in *Surgical Pathology*, Longmans Green, London, 1970.

Pauling, Linus, & Cameron, Ewan. *Cancer and Vitamin C: A Discussion of the Nature, Causes, Prevention and Treatment of Cancer with Special Reference to the Value of Vitamin C*, Warner Books, New York, 1979.

Pritikin Longevity Centre Newsletter, April 1976.

Queensland Fruit and Vegetable News, 18 September 1986.

Robinson, E D. Statement, National Biochemical Laboratory, New York.

Ross, F W Forbes. *Cancer: Its Genesis and Treatment*, Methuen, London, 1912.

Ross, M H. 'Proteins, calories and life expectancy', *Federation Proceedings*, vol. 18, 1959, page 1190.

Schweitzer, Albert. Cited in Max Gerson, *A Cancer Therapy: Results of Fifty Cases*, Totality Books, Delmar, California, 1958; distributed by the Gerson Institute, Bonita, California.

Science News, 9 September 1979. Report on the study in Holland showing that there was no reduction in dental cavities by the use of fluoride tablets or toothpaste.

Shamberger, Raymond. Address to the American Association for Cancer Research annual meeting in San Diego, May 1975.

Stamler, Jeremiah. Lecture on a study conducted by Loma Linda University, California, on Seventh Day Adventists, published in Circulation, July 1978.

Tipper, E H. *The Cradle of the World and Cancer*, 1927.

US Centre for Disease Control. Cited in *Fluoridation: The Great Dilemma*, Coronado Press, Lawrence, Kansas, 1978.

US Senate Select Committee on Nutrition and Human Needs. *Dietary Goals for the United States*, Government Printing Office, Washington DC, July 1976.

Vaccinations Condemned, Better Life Research, 1981.

Visek, Willard. Cited in Ross Horne, *The Health Revolution* (4th edn), Happy Landings, Avalon Beach NSW, 1985.

Voisin, Andre. *Soil, Grass and Cancer*, Crosby Lockwood, London, 1959.

Waldbott, George. *Flouridation: The Great Dilemma*, Coronado Press, Lawrence, Kansas, 1973.

Walker, Norman. *Colon Health*, Norwalk Press, Phoenix, Arizona.

Wattenberg, Leo. 'Inhibitors of chemical carcinogenesis', *Advances in Cancer Research*, vol. 26, no. 201, page 214, 1978.

Welles, William. 'The importance of squatting'.

Yiamouyiannis, J. 'Fluoridation and cancer', Fluoride, vol. 10, pages 102-23, 1977.

CHAPTER 8: UNCOMMON SENSE

Bell, Robert. *The Cancer Scourge and How to Destroy It*, Health Seekers International, Pinetown, South Africa.

Gerson, Max. *A Cancer Therapy: Results of Fifty Cases*, Totality Books, Delmar, California, 1958; distributed by the Gerson Institute, Bonita, California.

Gerson Healing Newsletter, 7 May 1994.

Haught, S J. *Has Doctor Max Gerson a True Cancer Cure?* (1962); later published as *Cancer, Think Curable*; later retitled *Censured for Curing Cancer: Dr Gerson's American Experience*, Gerson Institute, Bonita, California.

Kuhne, Louis. *The New Science of Healing*, translated from German, Williams & Norgate, London, 1894.

Moerman, Cornelius. *A Solution to the Cancer Problem*, C Moerman, Vlaardingen, Netherlands, 1962; English translation published by The International Association of Cancer Victims and Friends Inc., Los Angeles, 1962.

Sauerbruch, Ferdinand. *A Surgeon's Life*, Andre Deutsch, London, 1953.

Schweitzer, Albert. Cited in Max Gerson, *A Cancer Therapy: Results of Fifty Cases*, Totality Books, Delmar, California, 1958; distributed by the Gerson Institute, Bonita, California.

Warburg, Otto. 'The prime cause and prevention of cancer, with two prefaces on prevention', revised lecture of the meeting of the Nobel Laureates on 30 June 1966 at Lindau, Lake Constance, Germany' (2nd revd edn), English edition by Dean Burk, published by Konrad Triltsch, Würzburg, Germany, 1969. (Provided as Appendix A.)

CHAPTER 9: SPONTANEOUS REMISSION

Anderson, John. Cited in Peter Newton-Fenbow, *A Time to Heal*, Souvenir Press, London, 1971.

Chichester, Francis. *The Lonely Sea and the Sky*, Hodder & Stoughton, London, 1964.

Chichester, Francis. *Gipsy Moth Circles the World*, Hodder & Stoughton, London, 1967.

Ermer, Walter. *A Program for the Prevention and Early Detection of Cancer*, International Health Council Booklet no.110, Brea, Ohio.

Fredericks, Carlton. *Breast Cancer: A Nutritional Approach*, 1977.

Fredericks, Carlton. *Winning the Fight Against Breast Cancer*, Grosset & Dunlop, New York, 1977.

Gawler, Ian. You Can Conquer Cancer, Hill of Content, Melbourne, 1984.

Gerson, Max. *A Cancer Therapy: Results of Fifty Cases*, Totality Books, Delmar, California, 1958; distributed by the Gerson Institute, Bonita, California.

Gilford, Hastings. Cited in Cyril Scott, *Victory Over Cancer* (1939), Health Science Press, Bradford UK, 1974.

Haught, S J. *Has Doctor Max Gerson a True Cancer Cure?* (1962); later published as *Cancer, Think Curable*; later retitled *Censured for Curing Cancer: Dr Gerson's American Experience*, Gerson Institute, Bonita, California.

Hill, Eva, & Barrett, John. *Cancer and Cure: A Doctor's Story*, Bachman & Turner, London, 1976.

Issels, Joseph. *Cancer: A Second Opinion*, Hodder & Stoughton, London, 1975.

Koch, William F. *The Survival Factor in Neoplastic and Viral Diseases*, Vanderkloot Press, Detroit, 1961.

Le Shan, Lawrence. *You Can Fight for Your Life*, M Evans & Co, New York, 1977.

Luden, Georgine. Cited in Cyril Scott, *Victory Over Cancer* (1939), Health Science Press, Bradford UK, 1974.

Maxfield, James. Cited in Ross Horne, *The Health Revolution* (4th edn), Happy Landings, Avalon Beach NSW, 1985.

Meares, Ainslie. *Medical Journal of Australia*.

Medaris, John. Cited in Ross Horne, *The Health Revolution* (4th edn), Happy Landings, Avalon Beach NSW, 1985.

Newton-Fenbow, Peter. *A Time to Heal*, Souvenir Press, London, 1971.

Nolfi, Kristine. *My Experiences With Living Food*, 1954.

Quigley, D T. Cited in Ross Horne, *The Health Revolution* (4th edn), Happy Landings, Avalon Beach NSW, 1985.

Sattilaro, Anthony. *Recalled By Life*, Houghton Mifflin, Boston, 1983.

Sattilaro, Anthony. *Saturday Evening Post*, September 1980.

Schweitzer, Albert. Cited in Joseph Issels, *Cancer: A Second Opinion*, Hodder & Stoughton, London, 1975.

Scott, Cyril. *Victory Over Cancer* (1939), Health Science Press, Bradford UK, 1974.

Selye, Hans. *Stress Without Distress*.

Selye, Hans. *The Stress of Life*, McGraw Hill, 1956.

Simonton, O C, & Simonton, Stephanie. *Getting Well Again*, J P Tarcher Inc, Los Angeles, 1978.

Swanson, Gloria. Interview in *Here's Health*, May 1979.

CHAPTER 10: DIETING FOR HEALTH AND LONGEVITY

Densmore, Emmet. *How Nature Cures*, Stillman & Co, New York, 1892.

Evans, Charles De Lacy. *How to Prolong Life: An Enquiry into the Cause of Old Age and Natural Death* (1879), Charles Sawyer, London, 1910.

Gandhi, Mahatma *The Health Guide*, Crossings Press, Trumansburg, New York, 1965.

Garten, Max. *The Health Secrets of a Naturopathic Doctor*, Parker Publishing, New York, 1967.

Giese, Arthur C. *Living With Our Sun's Ultraviolet Rays*, Plenum Press, New York, 1976.

Horne, Ross. *The Health Revolution* (4th edn), Happy Landings, Avalon Beach NSW, 1985.

Horne, Ross. *Improving on Pritikin*, Happy Landings, Avalon Beach NSW, 1988

Howell, Edward. *The Status of Food Enzymes in Digestion and Metabolism*, National Enzyme Co, Chicago, 1946.

Howell, Edward. *Enzyme Nutrition*, Avery Publishing, Wayne, NJ, 1985.

Leaf, Alexander. *National Geographic*, January 1973.

Leaf, Alexander. *Youth in Old Age*, McGraw Hill, New York, 1975.

Lorand, Arnold. *Old Age Deferred*, F A Davis Co, Philadelphia, 1911.

Malisoff, William. *The Span of Life*, J B Lippincott Co, New York, 1937.

Palm, J Daniel. *Diet Away Your Stress, Tension and Anxiety*, Doubleday, New York, 1976).

Stamler, Jeremiah. Lecture on a study conducted by Loma Linda University, California, on Seventh Day Adventists, published in *Circulation*, July 1978.

Stiegbitz, Edward J. *The Second Forty Years*, Staples Press, London, 1949.

Williams, C J B. Cited by Charles De Lacy Evans, in *How to Prolong Life: An Enquiry into the Cause of Old Age and Natural Death* (1879), Charles Sawyer, London, 1910.

Wrench, G T. *The Wheel of Health*, C W Daniel & Co, London, 1938.

CHAPTER 11: IN CONCLUSION

Kenney, Joy. *The Pritikin Vantage Point*, vol. 4, no.7, July 1994.

New England Journal of Medicine, vol. 330, 1994, pages 1029–35. Report on a large-scale trial involving male smokers in Finland.

Warburg, Otto. 'The prime cause and prevention of cancer, with two prefaces on prevention', revised lecture of the meeting of the Nobel

Laureates on 30 June 1966 at Lindau, Lake Constance, Germany' (2nd revd edn), English edition by Dean Burk, published by Konrad Triltsch, Würzburg, Germany, 1969. (Provided as Appendix A.)

APPENDIX B: THE MEDICAL TREATMENT OF CANCER

Baum, M. *British Medical Journal*, 1976.

Bell, Robert. *The Cancer Scourge and How to Destroy It*, Health Seekers International, Pinetown, South Africa.

Blond, Kasper. *The Liver and Cancer: A New Cancer Therapy*, 1955.

Cunningham, L. 'Masectomy for so-called lobular carcinoma in situ', *Lancet*, vol. 1, page 306, 1980.

Dewey, W A. Cited in Maurice Natenberg, *The Cancer Blackout*, Regent House, 1959.

Goodfield, June. *Cancer Under Siege*, Hutchinson, London, 1975.

Horne, Ross. *The Health Revolution* (4th edn), Happy Landings, Avalon Beach NSW, 1985.

Humphrey, Hubert. Reported in *New York Daily News*, 14 January 1978; described in Ralph Moss, *The Cancer Syndrome*, Grove Press, New York, 1980.

Jones, Hardin. Lecture to the American Cancer Society's Annual Science Writers' Conference, New Orleans, March 1969.

Jones, Hardin. 'Demographic consideration of the cancer problem', New York Academy of Science, Series II, February 1956.

Paget, Sir James. Quotation from *Surgical Pathology*, Longmans Green, London, 1970.

Richards, Brian A. *The Topic of Cancer*, Pergamon Press, Oxford, 1982.

Shubik, P. Address to the Annual Scientific Meeting on the Subject of Cancer, Sydney University, November 1980.

Skrabanek, P. 'False premises and false promises of breast cancer screening', *Lancet*, vol. 2, pages 316-9, 1985.

APPENDIX C: THE DUBIOUS VALUE OF MAMMOGRAMS AND HORMONE REPLACEMENT THERAPY

Bassey, Joan. Study described in *New Scientist*, 23 October 1993.

Breslau, Neil A, et al. Article on the University of Texas Health Science Centre's research into diets rich in animal protein, in *Journal of Clin. Endo. Met.*, 1988, 140–46. Cited in *Pritikin Vantage Point*, July 1993.

Campbell, Colin. Cornell University study on eating habits in China, reported in *Pritikin Vantage Point*, July 1993.

Canadian National Breast Screening Study, findings published in *Health Freedom News* (Journal of the US National Health Federation), January 1995; also described by A B Miller et al., in *Canadian Medical Association*

Journal, vol. 147, no. 10, 1992; and in Stacey-Clear et al., *Lancet*, vol. 340, 1992.

Cooper, Kenneth. Lecture, 8 April 1995.

Hou, J, et al. Article on the University of California's research into diets high in fat and sugar affecting of bone density, in *Clin. Biomech.*, vol. 5, 1990, pages 162–8. Cited in *Pritikin Vantage Point*, July 1993.

National Cancer Institute (US). Report on the Breast Cancer Prevention Trial of the drug tamoxifen, described by Janet Raloff in *Science News*, 26 February 1994; also 'The tamoxifen scandal', *Health Freedom News*, May 1994.

National Health Federation (US). 'Do mammograms save womens' lives?', *Health Freedom News*, January 1995.

Vines, Gail. 'The challenge to HRT', *New Scientist*, 23 October 1993.

Singer, Frederick. *Pritikin Vantage Point*, vol. 3, no.7, July 1993.

Whitaker, Julian. 'Do mammograms save women's lives?', *Health Freedom News* (Journal of the US National Health Federation), January 1995.

Whitaker, Julian. *Reversing Health Risks*, Poseidon Press.

Whitaker, Julian. *Reversing Heart Disease*, Warner Books, New York, 1985.

Whitaker, Julian. *The Heart Surgery Trap*, Berkeley Publishing Group, California.

APPENDIX E: THE HISTORY OF THE PEDESTAL TOILET

Welles, William. 'The importance of squatting', *Natural Health Society Journal*, Penrith NSW.

List of further reading

CHAPTER 2: HEALTHY BLOOD, HEALTHY CELLS, HEALTHY BODY
Blood sludge
For further information, see Ross Horne, *The Health Revolution* (4th edn), Happy Landings, Avalon Beach NSW, 1985; especially Chapter 10, 'Blood viscosity as a factor in all metabolic diseases'.

Micro-organisms in the blood associated with various chronic pathological conditions
For further information, see Ross Horne, *Health and Survival in the 21st Century*, Margaret Gee Publishing, Sydney, 1992.

CHAPTER 5: SOME CANCER THEORIES
Diseases and vaccines
For further information, see Ross Horne, *Health and Survival in the 21st Century*, Margaret Gee Publishing, Sydney, 1992.

Diseases such as arthritis, asthma, diabetes and multiple sclerosis explained and successfully eliminated by natural means
For further information, see Ross Horne, *Health and Survival in the 21st Century*, Margaret Gee Publishing, Sydney, 1992.

The true causes of cancer, asthma, arthritis, heart disease, diabetes and othr 'diseases of civilisation'
For further information, see Ross Horne, *Health and Survival in the 21st Century*, Margaret Gee Publishing, Sydney, 1992.

CHAPTER 6: EXPLAINING CANCER
Anticoagulants
For further information, see Leopold Dintenfas, *Rheology of Blood in Diagnostic and Preventative Medicine*, Butterworth Press, 1976.

CHAPTER 7: MORE ON DIET AND OTHER FACTORS
Haemorrhoids
For further information about the squatting position, see BA Sikirov, 'Management of haemmorhoids: A new approach', *Israel Journal of Medical Science*, vol. 23, 1987.

Destruction of the immune system leads to AIDS
For further information, see Ross Horne, *Health and Survival in the 21st Century*, Margaret Gee Publishing, Sydney, 1992, Chapter 7, 'AIDS, yuppie flu and the common cold'.

Connection between immunisation and cot deaths
Archie Kalokerinos & Glen Dettman, *Second Thoughts About Disease*, 1977, and *Vaccinations Condemned*, Better Life Research, 1981.

Doctors with dissenting views on orthodox medicine
Robert S Mendelsohn, George Crile, Samuel Epstein, Henry Heimlich, Alan Scott Levin, Edward R Pinckney, David Spodick, Richard Moskowitz & George White, *Dissent in Medicine: Nine Doctors Speak Out*, Contemporary Books, Chicago, 1985. Essays in the book include: 'Immunisations: a dissenting view', 'How much science is there in modern medicine?', 'Corruption in American medicine', 'The inaccuracies of medical testing', 'Hospital births', 'Immunisations', 'Cancer treatment', and 'Environmental issues'.

CHAPTER 9: SPONTANEOUS REMISSION
Gerson therapy
The Gerson Therapy Primer, expanded and updated, for those wishing to know more about the Gerson therapy designed to assist the body accomplish the natural remission of cancer and other chronic complaints. Available from The Gerson Institute, Box 430, Bonita, California 91908–0430. The price (in May 1995) is US $15.00 plus postage.

CHAPTER 10: DIETING FOR HEALTH AND LONGEVITY
Problems encountered by eating cooked food
Explained in depth in Ross Horne, *The Health Revolution* (4th edn), Happy Landings, Avalon Beach NSW, 1985; and in Ross Horne, *Improving on Pritikin*, Happy Landings, Avalon Beach NSW, 1988.

Index